This book makes a strong case for better appreciation of the useful role of traditional African medicine in the health care service system and services in African countries. . . . My disagreements with some aspects of the book are due more to differences in our experience with traditional medicine practice and malaria research than in theoretical scientific concepts. The presentation is masterly in lucid stylish language easy to follow.

Professor Emeritus L. A. Salako
Department of Pharmacology & Therapeutics
University of Ibadan

This is a monumental study of the ideas, philosophies and science that constitute the heritage of traditional African medicine. This vast body of knowledge is often dismissed as superstition by the continent's neo-colonial elite. Yet the traditional African medicine is efficacious and ecologically relevant to Africa. This book adds to Professor Okpako's global reputation as an original Afro-centric scholar and thinker and will have an exponential impact on the theory of health and well being in Africa.

Professor G. G. Darah
President, Nigerian Oral Literature Association
formerly Nigerian Folklore Society

SCIENCE INTERROGATING BELIEF

Bridging the Old and New Traditions of Medicine in Africa

by
David T. Okpako

With a contribution from
Chukwuemeka Sylvester Nworu

and

Peter Achunike Akah

BookBuilders • Editions Africa

ISBN: 978 978 921 087 9 (cased)
978 978 921 088 6 (soft)

Published in Nigeria by
BookBuilders • Editions Africa
2 Awosika Avenue, Bodija, Ibadan
email: bookbuildersafrica@yahoo.com
mobile: 0805 662 9266; 0809 920 9106

Printed in Ibadan
Oluben Printers, Oke-Ado
mobile: 0805 522 0209

cover illustration

The cover image is Bruce Onobrakpeya's deep etching (1984) titled "Orakpo vore rinvwin muabo - a human wrestling with a spirit". It is used here with the permission of Professor Bruce Onobrakpeya and the Bruce Onobrakpeya Foundation, BOT©, with gratitude. The image captures the essence of the Urhobo emuerinvwin belief, discussed extensively in the book, which attributes serious illness of an unknown cause in an acculturated individual, to ancestor spirit anger or sustained wrestling with his/her conscience.

To Kath

CONTENTS

Preface. ix

Acknowledgements. xiii

Introduction. 1

PART ONE
The Enduring Value of Traditional African Medicine

1. Background to Theoretical Thinking in African
    Traditional Medicine: Definitions. 27

2. Traditional Asian and European Medicine. 41

3. Traditional African Modes of Thought
    and Scientific Theory. 49

4. Evidence that the Ancestor Spirit Anger Belief
    is a Metaphor. 81

PART TWO
The Organization of TAM Practices and the Concepts and Instruments Deployed in the Management of Serious Illness

5. Induction into the Healing Profession in
    African Medicine. 109

6. Specialists in the Management of Serious Illness. 117

7. Taboos and Witchcraft. 137

8. Herbs and Drugs as Therapeutic Tools: Pharmacology viewed
    from the perspective of traditional medicine. 153

9. Calabar Bean: A traditional African poison that
    yielded a famous drug. 169

Contents

10. From Poison to Drug: Examples of dramatic discoveries in Europe............................ 183

11. Speculations on the Origins of the Pharmacopoeia of Plant Remedies in Traditional African Medicine. 195

12. Dose of Medicine.................................. 211

13. The Placebo Effect................................ 221

14. Does Traditional Medicine Have a future in Africa?.................................. 239

PART THREE
Treatment of Minor Ailments in
Traditional African Medicine

15. Treatment of Minor Ailments in Traditional African Medicine: Malaria as a case study. 247

16. Treatment of Fever in Traditional African Medicine. ... 267

17. Inflammation and Malaria......................... 281

18. Drug Resistance in Malaria. 295

19. The Importance of an Africa-centred Approach to Malaria Control. 301

Afterword and Recommendations.................. 309

APPENDICES

Appendix 1:   Introduction to Chukwuemeka Sylvester Nworu & Peter Achunike Akah's Review. 325

Appendix 2:   Chukwuemeka Sylvester Nworu & Peter Achunike Akah: Anti-inflammatory Herbs and Their Molecular Mechanisms of Action. 329

Contents

Bibliography.. 359

Index. 363

PREFACE

Despite wide differences in practice details across the continent, certain key principles are identified which set traditional African medicine (TAM) apart as a distinct theory of healing, and not a rudimentary form of modern medicine: the beliefs that are deployed in diagnosis, prevention and treatment of serious illness in TAM, though not theories by strict scientific criteria, nevertheless derive from intuition, practical experience and observation, and encode important ideas that are critical to the understanding of the fundamental nature of illness. For example, the Africa-wide so-called ancestor spirit anger belief, which attributes serious illness (of indeterminate cause) to hidden sin (e.g., incest), that is forbidden by the ancestors, is shown in this study to be a composite of a metaphysical belief in the power of the supernatural to punish transgression, and experiential knowledge that the sinner's consciousness of his own misdemeanor is a factor in the occurrence of the illness. Ancestor spirit anger belief is therefore described in this book as metaphor for sustained emotional distress, and a return of an ill person to emotional equilibrium is a major therapeutic objective.

The esoteric methods, e.g., incantation, confessions, sacrifice, etc., used in TAM, which baffle the modern doctor, are in fact, procedures that diffuse emotional tension. They are not irrational superstitions.

In TAM then, a central theory is that serious illness has its origins in the mind; compare this with mind-body researches in modern medicine, (e.g. psychoneuroimmunology, PNI) which provides evidence that sustained emotions of fear, anxiety, anger, hatred, envy etc., can lower a person's immunity and predispose him to serious illness. Modern PNI theory thus grasps the essence of the ancient ancestor spirit anger belief. Other TAM beliefs, e.g. witchcraft and taboos, which also exploit the fear of supernatural punishment to control anti-social tendencies, are presented here as critical moral and health- related concepts in the African world view.

The fundamental difference between TAM and modern medicine is that in the latter, the germ theory of disease is the core paradigm, and elimination of a specific cause of disease is the treatment objective, whereas in the former, emotional stabilization is the major therapeutic objective in the treatment of serious illness. This difference explains, e.g., why rules of dosage in modern medicine need not apply in TAM; why TAM herbal remedies are derived from a pharmacopoeia of non-poisonous plants; why incantations in TAM and randomized clinical trials in modern medicine are "enhancers" of the placebo effect by different mechanisms, and why a search for drugs in TAM herbal remedies without familiarity with the core theoretical assumptions in TAM, is likely to fail.

The treatment of minor ailments (fever, aches and pains) is dealt with in the second half of the book. Minor ailments are commonly treated with plant-derived remedies which the people know to be effective for the purpose, without esoteric consultations, as we might use paracetamol without a doctor's prescription. Fever is probably the oldest symptom of disease known to man and diagnosed accurately by feel. Plant remedies that worked in alleviating it were known to indigenous people. Fever is a common symptom of malaria disease; it is also a quintessential manifestation of the biological phenomenon known as inflammation. Furthermore, it is now known that inflammation mechanisms account for many symptoms of malaria disease. Another remarkable convergence of science and African prescience intuition is the research finding in Nigeria in the last four decades that extracts of the plants used in TAM to treat fever, possess anti-inflammatory activity.

Combining the above observations, the following hypothesis is proposed: in prescience African societies, the symptomatic treatment of malaria amounted to a cure of the disease, because the people had substantial malaria immunity; suppression of the inflammatory symptoms by plant remedies caused a surge in immune activity and subsequent parasite elimination. This hypothesis is plausible considering that: (i) Africans survived in their malaria endemic regions long before modern malaria chemotherapy was introduced only about 100 years ago; (ii) many Nigerians still treat malaria/fever with plant-derived remedies, and what accounts for the success of such treatment is most probably, the anti-inflammatory, rather than any plasmodicidal (parasite killing) properties of the herbal remedies.

The idea that anti-inflammatory herbal symptomatic treatment is a cure for malaria disease in an otherwise healthy immunologically competent African adult living in a malaria endemic region is novel; the book suggests how anti-inflammatory herbal remedies can be recruited in the war against multi-drug resistance in malaria chemotherapy. Inflammation mechanisms are now known to initiate or enhance progression of many different chronic diseases in man, and the search is on worldwide for drugs that can act against a wide range of inflammation mechanisms. Plants possess an incredible array of chemical entities affecting different pathways of inflammation, not matched by synthetics.

The different experiences of the African people who have lived with malaria since the beginning of time, i.e., immunity and extensive knowledge of anti-fever plant remedies, should be factored into a suggested new Africa-centered approach to malaria control. The current strategy is inspired by Euro-American scholarship, ideology and funding, and is heavily influenced by European fear of malaria which earned West Africa, the terrible label of the 'white man's grave' in the 18th century. Its central plank is imported nets and drugs and it runs counter to the grain of the age-old biological equilibrium between man and parasite, and is not sustainable. This strategy should be tempered by injection of indigenous experience.

The book concludes with two recommendations: (i) Establishment of a National Centre for Malaria and Inflammation Research (NCMIR), and (ii) The principles of traditional African medicine should be taught in Nigerian Colleges of Medicine and Pharmacy.

ACKNOWLEDGMENTS

This work benefited from an eight-month residence as Visiting Fellow at the Humanities Research Centre, Australian National University, Canberra in 1996. I thank the then director, Professor Iain McCalman and the staff of the HRC for their kindness and generous hospitality, and for the opportunity to present several issues in this book at various conferences and discussions. I acknowledge the help and encouragement of medical anthropologist Dr. Margot Lyon of the ANC Canberra who introduced me to the literature on emotion and psychoneuroimmunology which helped me to understand and interpret the Urhobo concept of emuerinvwin as a shorthand expression of the critical association of immoral/anti-social conduct with serious illness.

I wish to thank my good friend and internationally acclaimed artist, Bruce Onobrakpeya, for allowing me to use one of his deep etchings "Orakpo vore rinvwin muabo - a human wrestling with a spirit" on the cover of this book.

I also wish to thank my colleague, Emeritus Professor L.A. Salako, a renowned malariologist and pharmacologist for kindly reading early drafts of the chapters on malaria and making extensive helpful comments. But needless to say, all remaining inadequacies and persisting controversial points of view are entirely mine.

Finally, I must thank generations of my students for inspiration and for helping to clarify some of the ideas presented in this book. I would like to acknowledge here that the three-day symposium to mark my 70th birthday anniversary titled Inflammation: An Underlying Factor in Several Diseases (unpublished) that was organized by former students in 2006, led by my first PhD student — M.A. Oriowo (Professor of Pharmacology, Kuwait University, Kuwait); Dr. (Mrs.) Yetunde Taiwo (Director, Global External Research & Development, Eli Lilly & Co., Indianapolis, USA);' Dr. A.S.O. Adeagbo (Associate Professor of Pharmacology, University of Louisville, Kentucky, USA); Sunny E. Ohia (Professor of Pharmacology & Dean, College of Pharmacy, University of Houston, Texas, USA); Janet Dupe Makinde (Professor of Pharmacology, University of Ibadan, Nigeria); Peter Akah (Professor of Pharmacology, University of Nigeria, Nsukka, Nigeria);Peter Aziba (Associate Professor of Pharmacology, Olabisi Onabanjo University, Sagamu, Nigeria — and many others, was a singular highly appreciated honour and an inspiration to write this book.

David T. Okpako
Akobo, Ibadan, May 2012

' Tragically, Dr. Yetunde Taiwo died of cancer in the USA in July 2012 while this manuscript was in preparation. My her soul rest in peace.

INTRODUCTION

Do the religious beliefs, taboos, incantations, divination etc., that are deployed in traditional African medicine, ostensibly, to prevent, diagnose and treat illness, have meanings relevant to health care as this is understood in modern medicine? Are they theories or are they ignorant superstitions? These are the sorts of questions that prompted this study. I must admit that I began with a bias, for at the back of my mind was the thought that if these beliefs collectively constituted the theoretical framework of the medical practices that sustained human life in Africa for millennia, there must be more to them than irrational superstitions. My starting point in this inquiry was therefore an attempt at interpretation of these beliefs, from my background of traditional upbringing in an Urhobo village, Owahwa in Delta State, Nigeria, and my subsequent professional experience as a biomedical scientist.

What intrigued me was the way traditional medicine practitioners in my clan, Ughievwen, used the Africa-wide belief that ancestor spirit anger can explain the occurrence of serious illness; that is, that dead ancestors can cause serious illness in an offending descendant who has committed an antisocial/immoral act known in Urhobo as emuerinvwin.

From the way the people deployed this belief in practice, it dawned on me that they knew, almost certainly from experience that, in an acculturated individual (someone brought up to know what kind of misdemeanor constitutes an emuerinvwin), the cause of a chronic illness is in the consciousness of the ill person. It seems that the ancients evolved ancestor spirit anger belief against the background of the knowledge that an acculturated individual who commits an emuerinvwin in secret would be emotionally distressed (ewen kpo kpo) and become ill if the sin was not exposed. In other words, the ancestor spirit anger concept is a composite of experiential knowledge and belief in the supernatural power of the ancestors to cause illness. It can therefore be understood as a metaphor for emotional distress arising from knowledge of a hidden sin. This became my working interpretation of the ancestor spirit anger belief.

My interpretation of beliefs in African medicine in this book is based on fieldwork and many years of contact with traditional medicine practitioners in one Nigerian ethnic community. But from a fair amount of reading of the literature on traditional medicine, I believe that the conclusions I reached from my study of this community in the Niger Delta, as to what constitutes the core theoretical assumptions about the causes of illness in African thought, are not exceptional but may be exemplary of traditional medicine processes in other parts of sub-Saharan Africa.

I have no professional training in the social sciences where fieldwork is a common tool of investigation. My approach to fieldwork was, therefore, rather informal and approximates to

what has been described as participant observation,[1] of traditional medicine methods in this part of Nigeria.

> Participant observation is a research approach in which the researcher becomes a spy of sorts. With disguised identity and interest, the investigator infiltrates the setting of interest and becomes a full-fledged participant in the group to be studied.

For me this was not difficult because I am a well known member of the clan/kingdom of Ughievwen, where the field work was done. In many cases, my participation in the traditional events (e.g., funerals) was mandatory as they involved my own lineage. My disguise was that I did not disclose my academic interest in the events or stories told to me at the time. In fact, the relevance to this work of what I experienced did not become apparent until I recalled them many years later, when I found that I could use the information in this study. Thus, I owe a profound gratitude to my kinsmen and women from whom I learnt a great deal about the culture, thereby making it possible to write this book.

It was somewhat reassuring to discover, in the course of the research for this book, that the essential elements

---

[1] R.B. Galdini, Influence,(Harper, 2007); Also see: Eva Giles, E. E. Evans-Pritchard, Witchcraft, Oracles and Magic among the Azande, (Oxford University Press, Oxford, 1976), p. 243.

of the ancient ancestor spirit anger belief, at least as I have interpreted it, are reflected in modern medical thinking: for example, research findings from psychoneuroimmunology or brain control of host immunity, an emerging specialty in modern medicine, provide evidence that sustained negative emotions of fear, anger, insecurity, grief, hate etc., can lower a person's immune activity and hence predispose such an individual to a variety of chronic debilitating illnesses.

Thus from a scientific standpoint ancestor spirit anger belief is a rational construct. All things considered, I came to the conclusion that in traditional African medicine (TAM) the basic principle around which all practices hover, is the knowledge gained from experience that serious illness in an acculturated individual has its roots in the mind, in sustained emotional distress, an idea that became crystallized as ancestor spirit anger belief; and, a return of the ill person to emotional equilibrium is a major therapeutic objective. This means that the esoteric procedures employed in the treatment of serious illness in TAM are, in fact, rational processes to diffuse emotional distress, not meaningless superstitions.

There is another dimension to this belief which merits reiteration. The belief has three elements which enables it to predict, explain and prevent the occurrence of serious illness:

I.   antisocial/immoral conduct by the ill person,

ii.   the knowledge of the power of conscience to

trouble the mind of an acculturated individual
as a contributory factor to illness, and

iii.   ancestor spirits (the supernatural) whose anger
is believed to trigger the illness.

It makes sense to suggest, as the belief does, that an
acculturated individual, who commits in secret, what he
knows to be an immorality liable to anger the ancestors,
will endure emotional distress due to attack of
conscience. The questions that can be raised however
are: What is the purpose of the belief? Did it evolve
solely for the purpose of making people ill? What
survival benefit, in evolutionary terms, could the belief
have conferred on traditional society? Are the ancestors
a group of egoistic supernatural beings who would not
brook a descendant's disavowal of their moral laws?
Such questions linger until we reflect on the significance
of good moral conduct and of immorality in prescience,
preliterate societies that had no centralized law
enforcement institutions.

In such small-scale kinship groups where,
presumably, the ideas encoded by the belief evolved,
what was a most critical requirement for group survival
was the harmonious relationship between its members,
so that they could act together to protect group interests.
The people, from years of experience, knew that certain
types of hidden immorality were inherently capable of
causing disharmony and therefore constituted a threat to
the cohesive survival of the group. Incest (the classic
example of emuerinvwin in Urhobo culture), for

example, has the capacity to cause havoc in interpersonal
relationships and to threaten the integrity of the group's
gene pool. In the absence of law enforcement institutions
as we know them today, to whom, but the incorruptible
supernatural ancestors and the individual's conscience,
could the people entrust moral lore enforcement, in
order to ensure social cohesion? In other words, the
ancestor spirit anger belief evolved primarily to preserve
the moral cohesion of the group. Serious illness was a
symptom that the sick person had committed an immoral
act that threatened the harmony and social cohesion in
the kinship. Its treatment, therefore, had to be holistic to
include relieving the sick person of his burden of guilt
thereby restoring him and the kinship group to
emotional equilibrium. At the same time the therapeutic
processes (divination, confessions and ritual sacrifices
etc.) acknowledged the crucial role of the ancestors as
enforcers of a strict moral code of conduct among
individuals in the group.

I have discussed this point at length in the text for its
importance on various grounds: first, it explains why
recovery from a serious illness was not the sole criterion
for judging success in traditional African medicine.
Consolidation of the moral integrity of the fragile kinship
group was also an important objective. One should not,
therefore, invalidate TAM treatment procedures simply
on the grounds that a seriously ill person may die even
after confessions and appropriate rituals have been
performed.

Second, concepts such as curse, taboos and witchcraft

which are regularly evoked in matters related to serious illness in TAM, all seem to exploit the active conscience of the acculturated individual: The fear that antisocial behaviour might ignite supernatural anger with consequent serious illness and possibly death, is a powerful deterrence against immoral conduct. These beliefs were rooted in the need for strict adherence to good social behaviour that guaranteed the cohesive survival of small-scale kinship groups.

These notions were not magic and they were not irrational superstitions. They survived in many African communities as explanation for the occurrence of serious illness. But, because the need for strict adherence to moral lore has ceased to be a way of life, and because we are ignorant of the survival imperatives that gave rise to them, modern Africans are hesitant, even ashamed, to defend these traditional concepts as deriving from genuine traditional African rational ideas about illness that evolved with positive purposes.

I have discussed these TAM beliefs at some length because they are examples of traditional African cultural practices which the educated African elite are under pressure to condemn and throw away, often without adequate inquiry as to their origins and inherent values. My conclusion overall is that in traditional African thought, serious illness is essentially a moral issue and a matter of conscience around which the different traditional African beliefs, concepts and practices have been woven.

This approach to the study of TAM, which also

attempts to explore the fundamental ideas that underpin the use of plant remedies in the system, has revealed an important fact that seems obvious but which has not been sufficiently articulated before now, which is that, there is a distinction between two levels of illness management in TAM: (I) serious illness that requires divination to unravel possible underlying spiritual causes, and (ii) minor or easy-to-diagnose ailments that are often self-diagnosed and self-medicated with commonly available medicinal plants without the need for esoteric consultations. In the treatment of minor ailments, where the cause of discomfort is self-evident, e.g., fever, aches and pains, efficacious TAM plant remedies are used just as aspirin would be used in the treatment of a headache in modern medicine. In my view, esoteric beliefs and concepts which are deployed in the management of serious illness, are given undue prominence by modern medicine in its negative characterization of TAM. In fact the common-sense use of plant remedies is the aspect of TAM that is most frequently practised by indigenous people.

That being the case, the subject of fever, a characteristic manifestation of a variety of diseases in which inflammation is an underlying mechanism, is extensively discussed in this book. Fever is an important disease symptom and must have been particularly so in prescience, preliterate societies; it can be determined without a thermometer by differential diagnosis (the body temperature of someone who is ill with fever being higher than that of a normal person), and this can be ascertained by touch. Fever was recognized by indigenous African healers as a sign of disease, and was treated effectively with herbal remedies. Fever was probably the only symptom of internal disease that prescience, pre-technology humans could identify with certainty. Coming closer to home, fever is a characteristic symptom of malaria. What indigenous Africans living in malaria endemic regions treated as fever almost certainly, included malaria fever, a problem that affected such people frequently. That is why we can assume that traditional herbal remedies were effective against malaria-induced fever. As matters have turned out in recent years, scientific research has revealed two remarkable coincidences:

I.   that inflammation is a critically important mechanism underlying the pathology of malaria, and

ii. that many of the herbal remedies used by indigenous people to treat fever possess anti-inflammatory pharmacological properties.

This means that Africans, though very likely unaware of the mosquito and plasmodium-parasitic origin of the disease, were successful at treating its symptoms. On this premise, I have put forward the hypothesis that such symptomatic treatment of malaria is tantamount to a cure of the disease in those people who are partially immune to malaria. I define partial immunity as consisting of naturally acquired immunity due to frequent contact with malaria parasite antigens, plus the various protective genetic adaptations which indigenous Africans living in malaria-endemic regions are known to possess.

If this theory is proven to have merit, it would mean a paradigm shift in our understanding of how to treat malaria in the partially immune person. It would also explain why malaria was not a killer of indigenous Africans on the same scale as native Europeans when first encountering the disease in West Africa in the early 20th century. The point is that the Plasmodium falciparum parasite develops resistance eventually to any plasmodicidal drug, i.e., any drug designed to kill it. It seems that the parasite does so in self defence and has done so for millennia.

Our experience of malaria chemotherapy so far bears out this scenario: any drug of this type, any plasmodicidal drug, sooner or later falls prey to Plasmodium falciparum resistance. Herbal treatment of malaria avoided a confrontation with the plasmodium parasite and therefore did not provoke it into deploying its considerable arsenal of drug resistance mechanisms.

This theory is at first sight controversial: We have been brought up to think that the only way to cure malaria is to kill the plasmodium parasite that causes it, but my idea can be tested in properly controlled preclinical studies and clinical trials.

The view advocated here is that all aspects of the African experience of malaria, including the extensive indigenous knowledge of anti-fever plant remedies, should be mobilized in the war against malaria. Unfortunately, this has not been done in a serious, concerted manner. We should do so if only as part of a search for alternative approaches to those dictated by conventional wisdom; the prescriptions handed down by expert committees from the World Health Organization (WHO) and sympathetic foreign donors, on how to deal with malaria have not always been the most appropriate; some may in fact run counter to the grain of biological equilibrium that existed between man and parasite in Africa before modern chemotherapy. In some respects, malaria seems to have become a far more dangerous disease since the new interventions.

I am placing emphasis on malaria in this part of the book to expose an even wider issue: Modern medical scientists have tended to ignore traditional African medicine as a source of ideas for healthcare in Africa, just as they have ignored other African traditional institutions; this is almost certainly because these institutions were denigrated, in the process of western colonial education. It is my view that the educated elite have largely upheld the European denigration of the African past, and have thereby indirectly contributed to Africa's woes; since independence from colonial rule, it is the educated elite, not traditional African institutions and their authorities, who have presided over the continent's drive towards so-called development; the results are there for all to see.

Traditional African medicine is one of the oldest methods of healing known to man, and probably goes further back in antiquity than the Indian and Chinese medicine traditions. In its various forms, TAM represents an important part of our heritage, embodying a most important body of indigenous knowledge passed down to us from ancient times. The view canvassed in this book is that this knowledge evolved to cope with the well-being of man in the African physical and cultural environment. The knowledge took millennia of African experience to accumulate and is ecologically relevant in matters concerning health in Africa. It is, therefore, imperative that the beliefs and symbols that go with TAM practices should be examined for meanings that may represent solutions to many intractable health problems in Africa.

Another reason why we must revisit TAM is that although the people of Africa have, in recent years, become exposed to other cultures through education and religious conversion, traditional medical beliefs have survived among a large majority of the people, many of whom now live in confusion in a world where those beliefs seem irrelevant to their health needs: consequently the people struggle to cope with modern medical theories and with TAM's beliefs, which often appear to be in conflict with each other.

So, they hedge their bets by patronizing both traditions — visiting both the diviner and the specialist hospital consultant, often simultaneously, with potentially dangerous consequences. I hope that this book will enable the modern medicine practitioner to understand the nature of the medical history that his traditional African patient brings to the modern clinic.

But the question can also be asked: Why bother to

study and write a book on traditional medicine in Africa now? After all, any new insights into human health in Africa that one may uncover from such an inquiry are already being addressed by science-driven advances in modern medicine. In any case, the most probable outcome of such an inquiry would be speculative—with conclusions and claims that cannot possibly be authenticated by ascertainable factual evidence. Would it not be better, therefore, to focus all efforts on how to improve modern medical facilities for the benefit of the African people?

From that standpoint, a serious commitment to the study of African medicine would seem an unnecessary distraction, or worse, an obstruction to modern medical progress in Africa. Why look back when it is obvious that progress lies in front?

This book represents a different view from the above argument which posits that TAM is a rudimentary form of modern medicine whose essences will in time, be subsumed by the latter. This book shows that such a view of TAM is simplistic or an outright fallacy. Simply from an ecological standpoint, ancient ideas on health and illness that took millennia to evolve in Africa, the crux of which have been distilled into beliefs and esoteric practices, demand a closer examination, for what they may be worth, for relevance to current African health needs.

Scepticism in some quarters is understandable. How does one evaluate TAM's significance as a healing method? Apart from the fantastic claims, anecdotes and myths surrounding African medicine, how do we know that TAM is rooted in ancient African rational thought? Unlike its Asian counterparts, for example, Ayurveda and traditional Chinese medicine, whose underlying philosophies were set down long ago in ancient manuscripts, TAM is an oral tradition. There is no generally accepted coherent basic principle, theory or philosophy on which its practices are grounded; only the beliefs and esoteric practices, some of which do not appear, on the face of it, to make rational medical sense.

This study provides evidence that the tag of mindless superstition placed on African medicine was unjustified. The description of TAM as such arose in an atmosphere of prevailing prejudices against virtually all African institutions at a time when some European thinkers even concluded that Africans had no language! The pioneers of modern medicine could not have considered the possibility that these so-called superstitions were shorthand representations of complex ideas and knowledge gained through experience and which might represent an understanding of the fundamental nature of illness. This book attempts to interpret these beliefs through the prism of current thinking in modern medicine in search of possible relevant meaning.

It was a mixed fortune that modern medicine, with its powerful science base and sometimes dramatic treatment successes, arrived in Africa at the time it did. The effect of modern medical theory was to discourage serious inquiry into TAM beliefs, myths and esoteric practices, which stood condemned as mindless superstitions. In the last one hundred years during which we have struggled to apply modern medicine models in Africa, the conditions of life that gave rise to TAM beliefs have receded into oblivion. In the prevailing environment dominated by foreign religious, science and technology ideologies, TAM beliefs have become irrevocably cast in the concrete of superstition in the minds of the elite; the further away we have 'advanced' from the type of traditional African communities in which TAM beliefs evolved, the harder it has been for the educated elite to see these beliefs other than as superstitions with little or no relevance to the health needs of African people.

My contention throughout this book is that the advances being made in the sciences actually provide new tools that we can use to explore the significance of ancient ideas on health in Africa. Disease diversity in human populations is ecologically driven: malaria is a good example. An interesting European example is cystic fibrosis (CF), a genetic disease that evolved as protective adaptation to cholera that devastated Europe in ancient times. Individuals who inherit two copies of the CF gene (one from each parent) suffer from CF disease characterized by trans-membrane chloride transport dysfunc-tion; whereas those who inherit one copy of the abnormal gene from one parent and normal gene from the other parent, are protected from cholera disease. The equivalent in Africa is the sickle cell gene that evolved as protective adaptation against malaria.

The different genetic and biochemical adaptations that people have had to make in order to survive diseases in their different ecological niches have resulted in differences in the prevalence and severity of various diseases among human populations: hypertension, diabetes and glaucoma occur at a greater frequency in people of African descent than in other populations, but the ecological bases of these have not been clearly defined.

Furthermore, the traditional management of diseases that are unique to particular ecologies comes from the experience and culture of the people in those environments. That is why the beliefs and esoteric concepts pertaining to illness and its management in Africa must be presumed to be rational and, ecologically and culturally relevant, and ought to be explored for their potential health benefits.

In 1976 the World Health Organization (WHO)[2], recog-nizing the potential contribution that traditional medicine can make to healthcare, convened a regional committee of medical scientists, bureaucrats and politicians with the aim of (I) defining traditional medicine and (ii) providing a framework for its exploitation as an additional tool in healthcare delivery in Africa. The committee came up with two definitions of traditional medicine:

> ... the sum total of all the knowledge and practices, whether explicable or not, used in diagnosis, prevention and elimination of physical, mental or

---

[2] World Health Organization (1976) African Traditional Medicine, Regional Office for Africa, Brazzaville, Afro Technical Report Series Number 1

social imbalance and relying exclusively on practical experience and observation handed down from generation to generation, whether verbally or in writing.

The other definition took note of the fact that traditional medicine was an 'amalgamation of dynamic medical know-how and ancestral experience'; hence TAM in particular was defined as:

> ... the sum total of practices, measures, ingredients and procedures of all kinds, whether material or not, which from time immemorial had enabled the African to guard against disease, to alleviate his suffering and to cure himself.

These two definitions of traditional medicine recognize the importance of the culture-derived esoteric evocations (ancestor spirit anger beliefs, divination, incantation, sacrifices, witchcraft beliefs and taboos) deployed in TAM, and the practical knowledge of the African pharmacopoeia of plant remedies used by traditional healers in the treatment of disease. The WHO paper was subsequently adopted as a working document by the Organization for African Unity (OAU).[3]

It is remarkable that only one of the committee's twelve recommendations on what actions African countries must take to increase the contribution of TAM to healthcare in Africa, stressed the need for a further consideration of the theoretical thinking that

---

[3] World Health Organization, African Traditional Medicine, Afro Technical Report Series Number 1 (Regional Office for Africa, Brazzaville, 1976).

underscores the use of plant materials in the system; that recommendation was "that scientific research be undertaken on the metaphysical aspects of traditional medicine". Unfortunately, little or no effort in that direction has been made in any African country since the recommendation was made. The result is that traditional medicine research in Africa in the last four decades has been synonymous with herbal medicine research to discover the active ingredients in plants used in TAM herbal remedies. The 'metaphysical aspects' of African medicine, that is to say, the theory behind the use of the herbal remedies have been ignored or ridiculed as superstitions.

The book is in 3 parts: Part 1 which comprises five chapters is my interpretation of health-related traditional African beliefs, namely, ancestor spirit anger explanation of illness, taboos, the curse, witchcraft, and divination and incantation practices, that are deployed in the diagnosis, prevention and treatment of serious illness i.e., life-threatening illnesses of unknown cause. When these beliefs and practices are examined in context in real situations of illness, we find that the ideas represent indigenous Africans' intuitive understanding of a critical association between serious illness and immorality, by which I mean, anti-social behaviour, that has the potential to undermine harmonious interpersonal relationships and therefore survival of the kinship group as a cohesive unit.

It seems that in traditional African societies, serious illness had a wider social significance than a threat to life of one person, as we tend to see illness in modern life. A serious life-threatening illness of unascertained cause was perceived as a threat to the existence of the kinship group as a harmonious unit. It was evidence of a grievous moral transgression by a member of the group that could, if not brought into the open for ritual treatment, cause disharmony and disintegration of the group. Therefore, cleansing the individual and the kinship group of the burden of the sin of immorality was at least, as important an objective, as curing the ill person. This holistic objective in African medicine is reflected in the elaborate rituals deployed in the management of serious illness including the characteristic unconventional (to modern medicine) methods of the use of plant medicines.

One of the scholars who has most influenced discussions of traditional African beliefs in the last four decades is the anthropologist, Professor Robin Horton of the University of Port Harcourt, Nigeria. His main conclusion is that such beliefs are rational in the context of African culture and, in some respects, are like theories in western science. Horton's work was an important point of departure for the theoretical aspects of this part of this book.

What I would consider to be my contribution to the debate is to point out that a short coming of many previous writings on traditional African beliefs is to discuss them from a western science perspective and then concede sympathetically, almost paternalistically that the beliefs are rational in the context of African culture. In contrast, my view is that traditional African beliefs, especially those relating to illness and its management, deserve analysis in their own right as theoretical constructs derived from ecological, evolutionary and environmental experience, not merely in abstract comparison with arcane Western scientific theories.

We also have to bear in mind that in traditional African thought there are no specializations such that one belief is exclusively about medicine, another about philosophy or sculpture, art, music etc. Virtually every traditional African belief or concept has, at its core, a religious configuration. Many great scholars including Robin Horton and Evans-Pritchard (of Witchcraft, Oracles and Magic fame), seemed not to take sufficient account of this characteristic of traditional African thought, leading them to the controversial conclusion that traditional African cultures are closed predicaments where there is no awareness of alternatives to established beliefs; whereas in Western scientific cultures such awareness is highly developed.

The fact is all religious doctrines are dogmatic closed predicaments: adherents of the faith do not seek alternatives to the dogma. This is as true in Africa as in the West.

Part 2 consists of 10 chapters: I describe concepts such as 'taboos', 'divination', 'the curse' 'incantations' and 'witchcraft' which are evoked in the management of serious illness (i.e., chronic life-threatening illness of an unknown cause). Here I make the point that although

TAM practices may appear to be characterized by informality and improvisation, certain common features can be identified that justify the use of the term traditional African medicine to describe the various methods of healing found in different parts of sub-Saharan Africa.

I describe the conceptual distinction between "serious and minor" ailments in TAM and why there are no organ or disease specialists in TAM, as we have them in modern medicine and this is due to the effect of the different theories of disease causation in the two systems. I draw attention to pharmacology in modern medicine as a theory in which drugs are deployed for the selective poisoning of the cause of disease; African herbal remedies in serious illness serve therapeutic purposes by mechanisms other than the selective poisoning of the cause of disease. It is in this respect that the differences between drugs in modern medicine and plant remedies in TAM manifest most profoundly: whereas dose regulation is imperative in modern medicine because the drug is a poison, such regulation need not apply in TAM, where the plants used are generally derived from a traditional pharmacopoeia from which overtly poisonous plants have been excluded.

Part 3 of the book has five chapters, in which I discuss the other important aspect of African medicine, namely, the use of herbal remedies in the treatment of minor ailments such as fevers, aches and pains, external bleeding, stomach upset, etc, that are often self-diagnosed and self-medicated without the need for esoteric methods which are deployed in the management of serious life-threatening illnesses. The treatment of minor ailments with commonly known plant remedies, without the doctor's prescription as it were, is the most widely practised form of traditional medicine. It is from the plant remedies used in this way that we should expect to discover medicines for the treatment of inflammatory diseases.

In writing Part 3 of the book I came to some intriguing insights from which I have made some challenging speculations. People in different ecological niches of the world historically discovered the plants that cured the diseases that troubled them most frequently; I suggest that it was the pressure from fever, the most widely recognized symptom of illness, that drove the autochthonous extensive knowledge of anti-fever plant remedies in African societies. Fever is the quintessential manifestation of the biological phenomenon known as inflammation, which is now known to be a major mechanism in the pathology of many diseases, including malaria. Thus fortuitously it would seem, traditional African communities evolved a pharmacopoeia of plants that possess anti-inflammatory properties, which they used regularly to treat malaria/fever, a disease that is currently considered to be basically an inflammatory disease. This convergence of African intuition and scientific evidence is remarkable; it is one reason why I advocate that the accumulated African experience of matters relating to health in this environment must not be ignored in the current war against malaria disease.

I will like to plead that if the readers of this book should find, for example, that in specific instances, their experience of African medicine practice in their own locality does not agree with some of my generalizations, I will not be at all surprised, given the unorganized nature of TAM. If the book provokes a constructive debate along these lines it shall have achieved a major objective.

I also appeal to the reader to approach the book with an open mind. Those of different faiths may find the many references to African traditional religion uncomfortable. Religion and medicine have been intricately intertwined in every traditional medical culture throughout human history. Africans were not different from other peoples in this respect. Furthermore, and as I pointed out already, African theoretical thinking tends to be holistic; there is no separation into specialties, such that one set of theoretical ideas is about medicine which is distinct from religion, sculpture, philosophy or science. All are connected and interrelated.

Finally, it is far from the intention of this writer to diminish in any way, the immense contributions made to the development of modern medicine in Africa by many great African medical scientists in many different specialties. In a sense this book is a tribute to their ingenuity to have successfully achieved what they achieved in an environment of two conflicting traditions. The aim in this book is to show that indigenous African thoughts on illness were rational outcomes of experience of life in the African environment and culture. It is my own way of apprehending the African past in the particular case of traditional African medicine.

*   *   *   *

PART ONE

SCIENCE INTERROGATING BELIEF

The Enduring Value of Traditional African Medicine Lies in the Methods of the Ancient Art

It does not enhance our understanding of African medicine by limiting ourselves to a search for drugs in the plants used in the system, dismissing the methods—incantations, divination and the like—as irrational superstitions. The real significance of traditional African medicine lies in these methods.[1] A substantial part of this book has thus been devoted to the interpretation of the methods. It encouraged me that a professor of medicine at Imperial College, London, told me he had included my short paper "Traditional African Medicine: Theory and Pharmacology Explored" published in Trends in Pharmacological Sciences (1999), on the reading list for his course on the subject: "Brain Control of Host Immunity".

---

[1] In a paper titled 'An ecological model of knowledge diversity' presented at the conference on Science and other Knowledge Traditions, in Cairns, Northern Australia in August, 1996, Professor Kai Hahweg (unpublished personal communication) drew attention to the following analogy: the Spanish conquistadores of the 16th century, not knowing the cultural value of the artworks of the Aztecs and the Incas in South America, melted the works down for the their metal – gold, silver and gem stones. The present day biomedical bio-prospectors, not understanding the cultural context in which plant remedies are used by traditional healers, melt down the remedies for their pharmacologically active chemical constituents. In both instances, the effect is to deprive indigenous people their cultural identity, and in the case of indigenous healers, to coerce them into accepting the framework of western science as superior to their own.

26

Chapter 1

Background to Theoretical Thinking in African Medicine: Definitions

D isease and death have been calamitous experiences of all human beings from the beginning of time. Therefore every society evolved ideas and practices for dealing with illness. These ideas grew out of each society's experience of illness in its particular ecological and cultural ambience on an evolutionary time-scale and against the background of the peoples' biological adaptation to the diseases that were prevalent and unique to that environment. Traditional African societies, where humanity thrived for thousands of years before the arrival of modern medicine only less than 500 years ago, were no exception. Indeed one might say that the earliest notions about illness and death first made their appearance in human consciousness in Africa.

The various forms of medicine practised in African communities today that are based on the peoples' experience of illness as passed down through generations by word of mouth, are what I refer to in this book as traditional African medicine or African medicine, or traditional medicine in Africa. The beliefs and esoteric concepts evoked as explanations of, and deployed in the prevention and treatment of illness, are what I refer to in this book as theoretical thinking in African medicine.

The World Health Organization[2] gives a broad definition of traditional medicine as:

> The sum total of all knowledge and practices, whether explicable or not, used in diagnosis, prevention and elimination of physical, mental or social imbalance and relying exclusively on practical experience and observations handed down from generation to generation whether verbally or in writing.

This thoughtful definition recognizes that traditional medicine practices are culture and environment bound (see below my brief references to the Asian medical systems). The medical anthropologist Professor Kleinman[3] describes medical traditions as "culture constructs". Accordingly, health and illness must be seen in broader socio-cultural perspectives than the narrow reductionist view of illness in biomedicine. He wrote:

> We can view medicine as a cultural system ... of symbolic meanings anchored in particular arrangements of social institutions and

---

[2] World Health Organization (1976) African Traditional Medicine, Regional Office for Africa, Brazzaville, Afro Technical Report Series Number 1; also see www.WHO.int/medicines/areas/traditional/ definitions /en (accessed 15 December 2014).

[3] A. Kleinman, Concepts and a model for the comparison of medical systems as cultural systems. in: Concepts of Health, Illness and Disease, Caroline Currer and Margaret Stacey, editors (Oxford, Bergamon Press, 1993), p. 42.

patterns of interpersonal interactions. In every culture, the response to it, individuals experiencing it and treating it and the social institutions relating to it are all systematically interconnected. The totality of these interrelationships is the health care system.

Professor Murray Last,[4] a University of London anthropologist who has studied traditional medicine practices in Northern Nigeria, uses the term medical culture in reference to 'all things medical that go on within a particular geographical area in which 'there exists a unique idiom, a subculture in which practitioners (healers and clients) can communicate and be mutually intelligible'. In African societies where traditional medicine is the dominant system of healing, the peoples' beliefs about illness derive from the same cultural experience.

Details in TAM procedures differ among countries in Africa, and even communities in the same country may differ in the way TAM is practised. Despite such differences, it will be seen in the course of the discussion in this book, that certain core principles can be identified which enable us to say that African medicine is a distinct system of healing, and why the use of the term 'traditional African medicine (TAM)' or 'African medicine' in this book is justified, even though the field observations on which this particular study is based were centred in one African community.

---

[4] Murray Last, The professionalization of African medicine: Ambiguities and definitions. in: The Professionalisation of African Medicine. M. Last and G. L. Chavunduka, editors (Manchester, Manchester University Press. 1986) pp.1-26.

Modern medicine which is now the dominant system of health care worldwide also grew out of indigenous ideas about illness in different traditional European societies, but modern medicine was built up cumulatively, a continuum from the past to the present, hence "the history of medicine" is a respectable field of scholarship among European scholars. In Africa, the educated class are reluctant to refer to Africa's past systems of thought, in particular, on matters relating to health and illness, convinced that traditional medicine practices were superstitions, in acquiescence with the European categorization of it as such in the colonial literature.

The fact of the matter is that the two forms of health care (traditional African and modern medicine) are practised in Africa. People move from one system to the other if their needs are not met. It is common for divination consultations to be going on outside the hospital on behalf of a patient who is under the care of modern medical specialists.

I have described one example of this from my fieldwork: Mr. O.O. had been ill and was admitted at the Ughelli General Hospital for what was diagnosed as congestive heart failure. Meanwhile, his middle-aged daughters from an earlier marriage, suspecting that there might be supernatural underpinnings to their father's illness had consulted an obo-epha (a diviner) who pronounced that their father's illness might be fatal due to a hidden abomination. Mr. O.O. was discharged after about two weeks, with digoxin and potassium supplement tablet prescriptions. O.O. died at home shortly afterwards. It came out at his 'postmortem inquest' that he had confessed to an abomination against the Ughievwen deity, Ogbaurhie.

Close relatives have been known to 'smuggle' traditional medicines into hospital as a result of divination consultations undertaken on behalf of patients, in order to supplement what the doctors are doing, to be certain that every eventuality is covered!

Many observations arise from these considerations: Modern medicine will continue to be the dominant healthcare system worldwide because of its strong scientific base and its ability to draw on a wide range of other disciplines and technologies to advance its frontiers. African countries must do their utmost to maintain the capability to keep abreast with these advances for the benefit of the people.

But there are some things that modern medicine in Africa must always keep in mind: Most of the patients and their relatives come from a background of traditional medicine and are imbued with ideas and attitudes internalized from the old practices. Such attitudes may hinder the optimal utilization of costly modern medical facilities. It is important that modern medical personnel should be aware of this fact so that they know when and how to apply the new knowledge to achieve the greatest good for the African. Given all that, why should the curriculum preparing doctors, nurses, pharmacists etc, who will administer health care to African patients, the majority of whom come from a background of traditional beliefs concerning illness, not include aspects of African medicine? An introduction to the basic principles of TAM would enable modern medicine practitioners to have some idea of the nature of traditional consultations taking place on behalf of the patients under their care.

The basic principles of TAM are embedded in the beliefs that are deployed in diagnosis, treatment and the prevention of serious illness, hence each belief needs to be critically analysed for meaning in the context of health care in Africa. The analysis of theoretical thinking in TAM is a major objective of this book.

Why there is no coherent TAM theory

One obvious reason that can be cited for this is that African communities were for long isolated from one another and the rest of the world culturally, physically and by language differences. While this could have been an impediment to the development of African medicine early on, it can no longer be a sufficient explanation for the absence of a coherent overarching theory in TAM. For the past 60 years or more, improved education and mass communication facilities, have brought African communities closer to one another and to the rest of the world. Isolationism is no longer a sufficient excuse for the absence of a generally accepted theoretical basis for African medicine practice. Other more fundamental reasons why African medicine did not develop a basic principle must include:

Historical impediments

Western-trained medical scientists do not usually take traditional African medicine, as a whole, seriously, either as an important subject for scholarly research or as a model of health care. To my mind, this is because early European explorers and subsequent colonial educators castigated TAM beliefs as superstition and of no value; the educated African elite seem to have accepted this view or could find no reason not to. On arrival in Africa, Europeans and their African collaborators instantly accorded modern medicine precedence over TAM. The effect of this indoctrination has persisted till today.

Early European explorers had come to the conclusion that the inhabitants of Africa were an inferior species of humanity, a view initially propagated to justify European exploitation of the conquered territories and their inhabitants, and was upheld throughout the colonial period. Unfortunately the tactics used by the European intelligentsia to denigrate African people and their traditional institutions became part of the imperial education and religious curricula which African people uncritically adopted. These European-derived institutions continue to be tools, even now, in the propagation of European models as the only way forward for Africa.

Traditional African medicine is a particularly cruel example of how successful 500 years of imperial education had been in turning the African, especially the western-trained African, away from serious engagement with Africa's traditional institutions. Admittedly, at the time of European arrival in Africa, Europe herself was just beginning to emerge from a period in her history

(see below for a brief sketch of early European thoughts
on medicine) when illness was attributed to even more
irrational and bizarre causes than the metaphysical
explanations they met in Africa. As Professor Adelola
Adeloye has pointed out in his important book, The
African Pioneers of Modern Medicine . Nigerian doctors
of the nineteenth century

> At that time, European medicine was still
> firmly in the grip of the miasmatic teaching
> which attributed human disease to the
> unwholesome influence of the elements.
> Treatment of diseases consisted of prosaic
> measures like purgation...and occasionally
> blood letting. Malaria, the dreaded fever which
> earned West Africa the frightening epithet of
> the "white man's grave" was thought to be due
> to emanation of foul air from decomposing
> vegetation, until the end of the 19th century
> when the malaria-mosquito theory was
> established. [5]

These early practitioners would not allow traditional
African explanations of illness to stand in the way of
medical progress; although they seemed impressed by
the large amount of herbal drugs used by the Yoruba
babalawo and onisegun, by the Benin and Urhobo ebos,
the Igbo dibia, the Efik mbia-ibok and Hausa mai magani
in different parts of Nigeria, but not by the theoretical
explanations of illness offered by these healers. Dr.
Oguntola Sapara who was familiar with traditional
medicine practices in Africa before going to study

---

[5] Adelola Adeloye, (Ibadan: University Press Ltd, 1985) p.38.

medicine in Scotland, became famous for his "Sapara's Children's Preserva-tive—Gbomoro" a concoction made from traditional herbs for the treatment of children's convulsions.[6]

The interest of these doctors in herbal remedies was not surprising, herbal medicines had commercial potential and the early medical curriculum in England and Scotland, where these pioneers trained, included the study of plant-derived crude drugs that were frequently used as therapies in the 19th and 20th century European medicine. These doctors were thus aware that plants are a source of curative remedies. But they were sceptical of the African fundamental beliefs, which, ironically, was like accepting the validity of drugs in modern medicine while at the same time denying the validity of the germ theory of disease. The lack of enthusiasm for indigenous peoples' beliefs concerning illness among African doctors dates back to this period. The effect of European contact was to discourage the educated elite from taking serious interest in the Africans' theoretical thinking in medicine. The development of TAM was thus aborted.

This was just one example of the general inhibitory impact that the European presence had on traditional African institutions. As Basil Davidson saw it:

> The whole great European project in Africa . . . can only seem a vast obstacle thrust across every reasonable avenue of African progress

---

[6] Ibid, p. 144.

out of preliterate and pre-scientific societies
into the modern world.[7]

In the view of Davidson, this contrasted with what
happened in Japan which, since 1867,

> . . . was able to accept westernization on its
> own terms, and its own speed... ensuring that
> new technology and organization were
> assimilated by Japanese thinkers and teachers
> without dishonor to ancestral shrines and gods.
> Japanese self confidence could be salvaged.
> Such an outcome was impossible in
> dispossessed Africa.[8]

The black educated children of former slaves, who in the
mid-19th century formed the vanguard of missionaries,
doctors and civil servants in the African colonies, also
had little sympathy for African cultural practices and
thereby confounded the problem. We learn from
Professor Adeloye that among the leading men who came
as doctors to West Africa were freed slaves or children
of freed slaves—the people Basil Davidson refers to as
"the children of the re-captives" who had had the good
fortune to study medicine in Europe. Davidson writes:

> The children of the re-captives reflected the
> full force of this alienation, for it was Africa,
> after all, that had consigned their parents to
> the damnations of slavery. [9]

---

[7] Basil Davidson, The Black Man's Burden–Africa and the Curse of the Nation-State (New York, Times Books, 1992) p. 42.

[8] Ibid.

[9] Ibid.

The point I am trying to make is that because early Europeans and their apologists saw no value in traditional African medical thought, the African medical scientists who succeeded them and who had been trained in European institutions, had no inclination to engage indigenous medical ideas, either as serious scholarship or as a model for the practice of medicine in Africa. The effect of European indoctrination still lingers, hindering an open-minded frontal apprehension of African traditional institutions.

Orality

One difficulty that can be cited as an excuse for the absence of a coherent principle in African medicine is that TAM is an oral tradition. The methods and thoughts underpinning African medicine practices have been transmitted from generation to generation by word-of-mouth. So that today every African traditional healer appears to be a law unto himself, interpreting and practising African medicine according to the tradition of his own lineage and often shielding certain aspects of the practice from prying eyes and ears. One consequence of the lack of a coherent basic principle in TAM is that efforts by various national authorities to systematize traditional medicine in Africa have failed to achieve the desired result, which is, to give traditional medicine a proper professional status in the health care delivery scheme.

Although orality has to be recognized as a problem when trying to analyse theoretical thinking in traditional

African cultures, experience from other fields such as African history and literature have shown that the oral tradition need not prevent an open-minded study of traditional medicine in search of a theory, if African medical scientists had had the intellectual inclination and drive to do so.

The limitations of the oral mode of transmitting theoretical thought through generations have been debated by social scientists in many volumes. We shall not go into those discussions here. Suffice it to say that the conclusion by Goody and Watt[10] (cited in Andah) that:

> ... among non-literate people (which to them is the same as oral) there can be no sense of continuous past or critical reflection of certain data concerning past events and acceptance of them; and its extension that critical approach depends on the ability to make use of written records and that on this also must depend the making of any distinction between history and myth.

This is a fair summary of the general view of unlettered people held by 'literate' societies: An event has to be written down and analysed for it to be history and, because what traditional non-literate people knew was not empirically derived, it could not possibly be knowledge. These views have been challenged by African scholars. The paper by Andah under reference is a good

[10] B.W. Andah, The oral versus the written word in the cognitive revolution: languages, culture and literacy. West African Journal of Anthropology (WAJA) Special Book Issue (20) 1990: 17-40.

example of such rebuttal. Furthermore, in the last several decades, African scholars have successfully established the validity of the oral approach to research in the African context, where it has been used to tease out whole swathes of African history and culture. In traditional medicine, core beliefs and practices have survived, despite orality; by a careful examination of these practices and beliefs, as I have tried to do in this study, it is possible to come close to the basic principles which underpin TAM practices.

Urgent health care demands

The pressure to deliver urgent modern health care in situations of inadequate facilities, which prevails in most African countries must be counted as an impediment to the exploration of meanings in African medicine. In such situations serious engagement with traditional medicine of the type necessary for the understanding of the fundamental assumptions behind traditional practices would seem to be an unnecessary luxury. Also, in the prevailing predominantly European culture in African medical colleges, those who want to progress in their academic and research careers cannot afford to devote effort to the study of a discipline (African medicine) that is unlikely to be of immediate application in the context of modern medicine. The results from such research would take long to come to fruition and are not likely to be accepted for publication in reputable medical journals. Most medical academics would cast such research aside because it would not come under the rubric of the overarching paradigm of modern medicine, namely, the germ theory of disease. There is at least one case to my knowledge of a brilliant medical physiologist whose promotion was delayed at the University of Ibadan because some of his excellent publications dealing with an aspect of traditional African medicine were not published in recognized journals of physiology!

Although there is no overarching principle around which TAM can be discussed, the system has survived modern medicine cynicism. This is a strong indication that in TAM, the practices are internally consistent with the assumptions it makes about the fundamental nature of illness and how to manage it. African practitioners of modern medicine intuitively recognize this, and therefore often adopt the paternalistic attitude of 'there may be something in TAM', but unfortunately, with little inclination to determine what that 'something' is. In the following chapters, I describe my findings which show that TAM beliefs and practices have underlying meanings that are relevant to health care delivery as we understand this to be in modern medicine.

Chapter 2

Traditional Asian and European
Medicine

C omparison is often made between African medicine on the one hand, and Asian traditional medicine, e.g., Indian Ayurveda and traditional Chinese medicine (TCM) on the other. Since the ideas underpinning Ayurveda and TCM practices, and their pharmacopoeias of plant remedies, are well-worked, having been set out in ancient manuscripts thousands of years ago, these systems, it is claimed, have an advantage in gaining the kind of universal acceptance that is denied traditional African medicine. Indeed, ideas derived from the Asian systems have found their way into western medical thought and practice: A notable example is acupuncture that has been incorporated into modern medical practice in different parts of the world even though there is still debate concerning efficacy and its mode of action. Ayurvedic colleges have been established in India where the principles of Ayurvedic medicine are being taught at the postgraduate level to doctors trained in modern medicine.

This is happening because scientists have more or less accepted the validity of some aspects of Ayurveda and TCM theories and are interpreting what were originally intuitively derived medical theories in the light of current knowledge in modern medicine: acupuncture has gained acceptability because of scientific evidence that it may operate through the nervous system; this is a modern interpretation of an ancient practice.

The availability of ancient documents gave the Asian systems a respectability which enabled modern medicine to learn something from the experience of these ancient Asians. There is no empirical proof of the scientific validity of every ancient idea that was expressed thousands of years ago in these documents, but antiquity and writing have endowed them with universal respect.

What I am saying is that even though ancient African thoughts on the cause of illness are not available as written documents, a careful analysis of the methods used by present-day practitioners can lead us to the core principles on which their practices are based. There can be some advantage in this. Our interpretations would be based on deductions made from the practices of TAM healers in the light of prevailing biomedical theories, and would not be constrained by ancient dogmas in divine manuscripts.

Ayurveda, TCM and TAM are probably the oldest traditional healing methods in the world today patronized by large numbers of people. This seems a good place in this book to briefly describe the basic principles of the Asian systems, and to say a few words about early European medicine in order to put modern medicine in perspective. And then when we come to working out the basic principles of TAM, not from manuscripts, but from deductions made from a close scrutiny of what practitioners of TAM actually do, it will be seen that all people (Africans, Europeans and Asians) had similar intuitive understanding of what lies behind human illness.

Ayurveda[11]

The earliest concepts of Indian medicine are set out in the sacred writings called Vedas and date as far back as the second millennium B.C. All later writings on Indian medicine are said to be based on these early concepts. According to Ayurvedic theory,[12] the human body consists of three elementary substances (doshas) which are microcosmic representatives of three divine universal forces: spirit (vata), phlegm (kapha) and bile (pitta). It is believed that there is a complex relationship between these three elementary substances and the physiological functions of the human body in health and disease. The doshas also control emotion and behaviour. Disease or proneness to disease occurs if there is imbalance of the three doshas, and restoration of their equilibrium eliminates disease. In Ayurveda, treatment is aimed, not only at curing the disease but also at enhancing the body's capacity to prevent the recurrence of disease. Ayurveda is described as the science of longevity and

---

11 This description is based on M. Thomas, "The Ayurvedic System of Medicine", in: Principles of Pharmacology: Tropical Approach, second edition, DT Okpako, editor (Cambridge, Cambridge University Press, 2003) p. 4.

12 G. Obeyesekere, The theory of psychological medicine in the ayurvedic tradition, Culture, Medicine and Psychiatry 1977; (1): 155-81.

positive health; it epitomizes the philosophy of total healthcare, the patient as a whole is given attention. Thus Ayurveda is not merely a medical science but a way of life.

Indians believe that Ayurveda was born out of intuition and divine revelation. In Ayurvedic theory,[13] physical health is maintained when the three doshas are in harmonious balance. When any of the doshas is out of balance, illness results, when all three are upset, serious illness results. The aim of therapy is therefore to reduce or control the excesses of an overactive dosha and to restore the system to a state of equilibrium.

Traditional Chinese Medicine [14]

In traditional Chinese medicine (TCM) the concept of harmony is central to well-being. The theory is that illness results from an imbalance in the elaborate opposites which are called yin and yang (positive and negative forces). Illnesses are therefore categorized as to what yin or yang element is out of tune (cf. the doshas in Ayurveda). The aim of therapy is to restore the patient to a harmonious relationship by various methods including the use of plant remedies that are deemed to possess the appropriate yin or yang corrective properties.

Traditional European medicine

---

13 Ibid.

14 E. P. Y. Chow, "Traditional Chinese Medicine: a holistic system", in: Alternative Medicines, Popular and Policy Perspectives, W. Salmon, editor (New York & London: Tavistock 1984).

Early European medicine can be traced to Hippocrates in the fourth centuryB.C. but it was Galen (A.D.131-200) who formalized the system of medicine that was practised in Europe for 1500 years.[15] Galen's main theory was that the

> . . . state of bodily health was preserved by the presence, in their proper proportions, of the four humours: heat, cold, dryness and moisture. Disease was supposed to result from a disturbance in balance of these humours, and the disease could be cured by an administration of various drugs possessing these fundamental qualities.

In Galen's theory we see the resonance of the older traditional Asian and African ideas of harmony as critical requirement for good health. Galen's theories held sway until the 16th century A.D., when the teachings of Paracelsus (Theophrastus von Hohenheim, born 1493), also famous for his formulation of the doctrine of signature took over. Much of Paracelsus medical theory was overlaid with a nonsensical mass of astrology, mysticism and alchemy.[16]

It was not until the late 19th century after a number of scientific methods had been introduced into medical practice did the germ theory of disease emerge. Discoveries by the great European scientists such as Pasteur, Lister, Koch and Ehrlich led ultimately to the

---

15 T.S. Work and E. Work, The Basis of Chemotherapy (Edinburgh, Oliver and Boyd, 1948) p.3.

16 Ibid.

universal acceptance of the germ theory of disease, which is that, diseases are caused by microscopic organisms invisible to the naked eye, called germs. This was when European medicine began to turn away from the 'nonsensical mass of astrology, mysticism and alchemy' that characterized medicine up till then.

These developments were greatly helped by advances in technology. The microscope enabled scientists to see germs and study them; weights, volumes and time could be measured accurately in absolute units. Precision measurements critically contributed to the progress of modern medicine since the 19th century. Specifically, developments in precision technology enabled poisonous substances to be used successfully as drugs in the treatment of disease.

Why the management of serious illness in traditional medicine is holistic

The critically important idea that to be in good health, a person must be in harmony with the natural environment seems to have been part of theoretical thinking in traditional medicine from the beginning of human existence. The Ayurvedic theory speaks of the need for the doshas to be in equilibrium as a requirement for good health. Emotional stress e.g. anger, fear, greed, infatuation, excitement, grief, worry, anxiety, can upset the doshas and cause illness.

In traditional Chinese medicine, it is the balance in the complex opposites, yin and yang, which must be maintained for good health to prevail. Herbal remedies are used to address a yin and yang imbalance. Traditional European medicine had similar thoughts expressed in terms of the balance of the humours. The idea of harmony with nature as a requirement for health, for the absence of illness, is an autochthonous idea that evolved with humanity in different parts of the world.

In African medicine the idea of harmony with nature as a requirement for good health is also of vital importance. For the African, nature includes not only the physical environment but also the unseen world of the gods and the spirits. Professor T.A. Lambo, the great Nigerian psychiatrist and one time deputy director-general of the World Health Organization expressed the African world view in this regard succinctly as follows:

> All living things including man are linked in harmonious relationships with the gods and the spirits, so that reality consists in the relation, not of man with things but of man with man and of all with the spirits.[17]

The African idea of harmony with nature as a requirement for good health is expressed most profoundly in the Urhobo belief in emuerinvwin in which illness, especially serious life-threatening illness, is ascribable to the anger of the ancestors.

The imperative for a harmonious relationship between a person and the natural environment for good

---

[17] T.A. Lambo, Traditional African culture and western medicine, in: Medicine and Culture, F N Poynter, editor, (London, Wellcome Institute of the History of Medicine, 1969).

health is what drives the holistic approach in all traditional healing systems. Holistic treatment means that therapy is directed at the whole person, not merely at the disease; the aim is to enable the body to heal itself.

This brings to mind a criticism that has been levelled against modern medicine: that modern medicine has the tendency to 'fight the disease' almost to the neglect of the person harbouring it, because of the tendency to assume a mind-body dichotomy in modern medicine, and illness is treated with almost complete disregard to the patient's personal insight into its cause and what to do about it. What technological diagnosis uncovers as the cause of illness takes precedence over any other consideration. Science and technology have imposed themselves between man and his need for harmonious relationship with nature. But S & T have not solved all health problems and there is increasing evidence that sustained emotional turmoil can lead to physical illness. It is thus an appropriate time to have another look at the old beliefs in traditional African medicine (TAM).

Chapter 3

Traditional African Modes of Thought
and Scientific Theory[18]

A ll over Africa, south of the Sahara, indigenous people evoke supernatural explanations for the occurrence of serious life-threatening illness or death or other misfortune; for example, it is believed in many parts of Africa that dead ancestors can inflict serious illness or death on someone who has angered them in some way, and that ritual sacrifices aimed at propitiating the ancestors can bring about healing in such illnesses. This is usually referred to as ancestor spirit anger belief.

It is the kind of thinking that leading sociologists of the early 20th century, notably Levy-Bruhl and Emil Durkheim, described as primitive or preliterate modes of thought, which they claimed could be distinguished from the Western or scientific way of thinking. Primitive and western scientific ways of thinking were considered

---

18 The substance of this chapter was first given as the Sir Kashim Ibrahim Memorial Lecture under the auspices of the Nigerian Academy of Science with the title, "How Do We Know? Reflections on theoretical thinking in traditional African medicine"; and in: D.T. Okpako, Malaria and Indigenous Knowledge in Africa, (Ibadan: Ibadan University Press, 2011) Some elements in that paper are reproduced here with permission.

to be radically different from one another and that the primitive man can only think like the western man by a process of 'inversion', that is, by abandoning the primitive mode, from which it is impossible to progress to the western scientific mode.

The reasons for this were put down to various emotional needs of people living in closely-knit groups and the fact that collective representation (e.g. kinship group collective beliefs) in small scale societies did not allow for individual reasoning. Primitive thinking was thought to be essentially mystical, and primitives were regarded as being indifferent to consistency of ideas. Therefore, according to these writers, rationality was not the key to understanding such beliefs.[19]

This study shows (see below in this chapter) that the above is an oversimplification; in at least in one case, namely, the ancestor spirit anger explanation of illness, there is evidence that the belief is a composite of two ideas: on the one hand, knowledge from experience that an acculturated individual harbouring knowledge of guilt would have a gnawing conscience; and on the other, the belief that a resulting illness is an affliction of angered ancestors. The belief can thus be understood as a shorthand reference to sustained emotional distress, which I contend, the people knew from experience to predispose to serious illness. The ancestor spirit anger explanation of illness is therefore, not an irrational belief but a distillate of accumulated experience.

---

19 R. Horton, Levy-Bruhl, Durkheim and the scientific revolution, in: Modes of Thought—Essays on Thinking in Western and non-Western Societies, Robin Horton and Ruth Finnegan, editors, (London: Faber & Faber, 1973).

Understanding the belief as the essence of accumulated experience of the relationship between immorality and serious illness, enables us to treat the belief as a scientific proposition, for example, in relation to the theory in psychoneuro-immunology, that the brain exerts significant control on a person's immune activity. Once this insight was grasped, a major challenge in this study, was to see if there was evidence for such a view from the way traditional healers and their clients deployed the belief in real instances of serious illness; the evidence supports the theory that ancestor spirit anger belief is indeed a shorthand reference to sustained emotional upheaval; then the logic of many of the practices in TAM (incantation, divination, confessions, etc) hitherto considered 'inexplicable, fell into place.

Furthermore, the notion that human beings could be differentiated on the basis of how they think, not the content of the thought, has been criticized by many writers. In the first place[20] Wiredu argues that it is unhelpful to compare pre-scientific traditional African thought patterns with modern western science. What would be interesting, according to Professor Wiredu, would be a cross-cultural comparison between pre-scientific traditional African thought, and western thought at the same level of development when both societies were driven by similar concerns (e.g., compare Galen's theories of medicine in 12th century Europe with ancestor spirit anger explanation of illness in African medicine in the last chapter). One consequence of comparing preliterate traditional African thought with

---

20 K. Wiredu, Philosophy and an African Culture (Cambridge, Cambridge University Press, 1980) p. 39.

western science is that many westerners have gone about with an exaggerated notion of the differences in nature between Africans and other people.[21]

A professor of philosophy (University of Ibadan), Godwin Sogolo[22] goes further to say that it is futile to attempt to categorize people in this way; "any attempt to lay down some specific criteria by which a traditional thought is to be distinguished from a modern one is not only problematic but misguided".

The insistence by some of these early writers that religious beliefs were characteristic of preliterate modes of thought was also a problem. According to Morris [23]

> . . . by focusing largely on their religious conceptions, Levy-Bruhl made the mental world of preliterate people seem more mystical than it really was. He portrayed preliterate people as living continuously upon the mystical plane, whereas in fact they spent much of their time at the level of common sense where the Western ethnographer would be able to communicate with them without any difficulty.

These criticisms are valid: If the ethnographer was to inquire from the African dugout canoe builder why the canoe floats on water, the latter would not, in all probability, not offer a supernatural explanation; he would not likely evoke Archimede's Principle as

---

21 Ibid.

22 Godwin Sogolo Foundations of African Philosophy - A definitive analysis of conceptual issues in African thought. (Ibadan, Ibadan University Press, 1993) p. 41.

23 B. Morris, Anthropological Studies of Religion: An introductory text, (Cambridge, University Press, Cambridge, 1995) p. 185.

explanation either, but neither would the ordinary Englishman in a London street nor even the ordinary English labourer in a ship building dockyard! Not all everyday activities of Western man are consciously guided by arcane scientific thinking; neither does the traditional African person evoke the spirits in his every day activities.

In accordance with traditional African beliefs and medical practices, the evocation of ancestor spirit anger, the use of divination as a diagnostic mechanism and the recitation of the appropriate incantation as an essential therapeutic procedure are consistent with the practical objective of restoring a seriously ill patient to a state of emotional equilibrium, the theory being that serious life-threatening illnesses have their origins in sustained emotional distress.

Ancestors and ancestor spirit anger are big ideas
in African medicine

Belief in the existence of the spirits of dead ancestors and the influence on the lives of their descendants has existed among human populations from time immemorial. In particular, the belief that dead ancestor spirits can cause serious illness in those who fail to adhere to moral laws laid down by the ancestors, is widespread in sub-Saharan Africa and in virtually every ethnic nationality in Nigeria.[24] This belief is among the

---

24 See for example, Ghana: P.A.Twumasi, Medical Systems in Ghana- A study in medical sociology (Tema, Ghana Publishing Corporation , 1975) p. 37; Congo: J.M. Janzen,The Quest for Therapy: Medical pluralism in the Lower Zaire. (Berkeley, University of California Press,1978) p.158; Tiv, Nigeria: D.R. Price-Williams, A case study of ideas concerning disease among the Tiv. in: African Therapeutic Systems. Z.A. Ademuwagun, J. A.

most frequently encountered as explanation for the
occurrence of serious illness in TAM. I consider it to be
the central idea around which all the various practical
processes in TAM hover, especially in regard to the
management of serious illness.

Belief in the reality of the spirits of dead ancestors is
more widespread among human beings than is generally
realized. According to Fraser[25] the belief is a reflection
of the almost universal belief in the survival of the
human spirit after death —a belief so flattering to human
vanity and so comforting to human sorrow that it has
survived in different societies in different forms. In
ancient Egypt[26]

> The concept of after life was originally limited
> to royalty. In time however, the nobility and
> privileged classes came to have hope of
> attaining the same kind of eternal existence. By
> the New Kingdom such access was within reach
> of even more of the population. To qualify for
> entry into an eternal existence one had to have
> lived an exemplary life on earth.

As noted below among Ughievwen/Urhobo, the world of
the ancestors consists of more than one domain; the
highest domain (erinvwin), where the moral laws that
govern conduct among descendants are made and

A. Ayoade, I. E. Harrison and D. M. Warren, editors, Boston, Cross Roads
Press, 1979) p. 158; Zambia: V. Turner, Drums of Affliction - A study of
religious processes among the Ndemu of Zambia. (London, IAP
Hutchinson University for Africa, 1981)p. 61-62.

25 J.G. Fraser, The Fear of the Dead in Primitive Religion, (London,
Macmillan & Co. 1933) p. vi.

26 D.P. Silverman, Divinity and Deities in Ancient Egypt, in: Religion in
Ancient Egypt, B. E. Schafer, editor, (London, Rutledge, 1991) p. 46-47.

enforced, is inhabited by the highest ranking ancestors, that is, those who lived exemplary lives while in this world. Others who did not live fulfilled lives, who died young, or of dangerous diseases, or were criminals etc., are treated with less reverence as the lesser erinvwin.

For example during Ore, the Ughievwen festival of the ancestors, the head of the kinship group offers with the left hand, the libation to the lesser erinvwin who are called upon to partake of the offering outside the ancestral shrine of the kinship group. This is indicative of Ughievwen/Urhobo classification of ancestors into two categories: the lower deserving of less reverence than the higher who must partake of the libations offered to them by the right hand and at the ancestral shrine, somewhat reminiscent of the ancient Egyptian hierarchical categorization of those who could attain eternity after death. It is also interesting to compare the Ughievwen practice whereby the lesser erinvwin must partake of the libation offered to them outside the ancestral shrine, with the traditional practice among the Karens of Burma where, according to an 1888 account cited by Fraser[27]

In fear of the ghosts of the dead, the people go to the forest and there deposit a little basket of coloured rice saying: "ghosts of those who died by falling from a tree, ghosts of those who died of hunger or thirst, ghosts of those who died of a tiger's tooth or a serpent's fang, ghosts of those who perished of cholera or small pox, ghosts of those who died of leprosy, do not molest us, do not catch us, do not do us any harm. Stay here in the woods. We will take care of you; we will bring you red, yellow and white rice for your subsistence".

---

27 Fraser, op cit.

It is tempting to speculate that ideas of this sort could have diffused from ancient Africa into Egypt, and dispersed from there to other parts of the world. Be that as it may, it would appear that the belief in life after death which underpins the belief in ancestor spirits has existed in different cultures of the world from the beginning of time.

Ancestor veneration is the core of Ughievwen traditional religion

My memory of the religious life when growing up in my home village of Owahwa was principally of the annual celebration of the feast of the ancestors called Ore, one day for the male ancestors (ose re emo) and another day for the female ancestors (oni re emo). The clan deity under whose umbrella the veneration of the ancestors took place is Ogbaurhie (the powerful one of the river). Owahwa town is the headquarters of the subclan of that name in the Clan Kingdom of Ughievwen, one of the 23 or so kingdoms that make up the Urhobo ethnic nationality of Delta State, Nigeria.

The Ogbaurhie shrine is located at Otor-Ughievwen, headquarters of Ughievwen Kingdom. Some Christian sects condemn the Urhobo veneration of their ancestors as idol worship and unChristian, which has resulted in an almost total cessation of the Ore festival in Ughievwen land.

The Ughievwen annual Ore is a feast of remembrance, to honour and venerate the ancestors. Reverend Father Monsignor Anthony Erhueh makes the point that the Urhobo do not worship their ancestors but venerate them just as people everywhere do one way or another.[28]. The Urhobo believe that the Almighty God, the creator of the universe is Oghene. Ancestor veneration is based on the interplay between the living and the dead, that is, communion between one's family past, present and future. Ancestor veneration shows that what is done on earth has significance for eternal life; that death does not actually sever the family bond, that man's actions affect the whole human family, living and dead; and finally, that man is immortal as a person, and therefore, he is the image of God.[29] I have cited this authority to show that the Urhobo are an African traditional society where the belief in the influence of ancestors in the life of their descendants is formalized as a religious institution.

The Ughievwen Clan Kingdom has an estimated number of more than 30 towns and villages and more than 200,000 people, who have been relatively isolated from Western influence. I investigated TAM practices by observation and direct interviews. Until the advent of various Christian denominations in the last four decades, traditional religious beliefs such as the belief in the influence of dead ancestors in the affairs of their living descendants, governed the way people in this community conducted themselves when faced with serious illness in one of their members. And, despite Christian influence, this belief is still widely held by the Urhobo generally.

In my village (Owahwa) it does not take much probing for the strength of this belief to manifest even among those who are Christian converts.

---

28 A.O. Erhueh, Vatican II: Image of God in Man. (Urbaniana University Press, Rome, 1987)p. 260-273.

29 Ibid., 273.

The belief in ancestors is given practical expression in the form of highly structured public celebration, veneration and festivals. Erinvwin is the mental space inhabited by the people who are dead to the living descendants. It is clear from the way Ughienvwen offer libation to their ancestors, as described above, that the people have in mind more than one category of dead ancestors inhabiting different spatial locations in the world of the dead. High erinvwin is the domain of dead ancestors of high integrity, men and women who wielded moral authority while they were alive, and remain even after their death, the custodians of moral law among their descendants; their abode is, shall we say, not far from the homesteads of their descendants, but separate from the imaginary abode of the lesser erinvwin consisting of dead criminals, witches, sorcerers, those who died of dangerous diseases or suicide, or who were insane, i.e., men and women who could not lay claim to moral authority or community leadership while they were alive, people who were not buried in their own homes or were considered unfit to be buried among the descendants.

Concept of emuerinvwin

The belief in the influence of ancestors plays an important role in ensuring adherence to critical moral laws in traditional Urhobo society; if a moral law is breached, only the ancestors can be trusted to determine what sanctions are appropriate for an offender. Such wrongdoings are thus known as emuerinvwin (literally a matter for the ancestors).

Incest which is broadly interpreted to mean sexual intercourse between a man and a woman for whom a blood relationship can be traced such as cousins, even if they are several times removed, extra-marital intercourse by a married woman, intercourse between a man and the wife of a blood relative, etc., are all typical emuerinvwin in Urhobo moral lore. It is pertinent to note that other types of antisocial conduct, e.g., theft, graft, deceit, male adultery, bribery and corruption etc, are not emuerinvwin, unless the act was committed against kin. Other methods are available for dealing with such behaviour.

Incest is serious abomination forbidden by erinvwin; its commission is a threat to the social cohesion of the community. Hence only the ancestors of high integrity can be trusted to impartially award punishment for such a sin. The fear of erinvwin sanction which may be serious illness or death is so potent that social contact between the sexes in the kinship unit in traditional Urhobo society is carefully monitored, everyone has to be sure not to get too carelessly close to the opposite sex in the kinship group. Assigning judgement in matters concerning the contravention of moral laws that threatened society's harmonious cohesion to high ranking ancestors was a wise move. The ancestors could not be lied to, and they could not be bribed! Their judgement could not be challenged

The Urhobo think of the ancestors as being dead to the living but alive in Erinvwin; they do not think of their dead ancestors as 'spirits' but as people just as they were when they were alive. In libation, the individual ancestor is addressed by name, not as a spirit. Scholars such as Michael Nabofa and John Mbiti use the term 'the living dead' to describe ancestor spirits. Although I use the term 'ancestor spirit anger' in this discussion I have in mind the view of the Urhobo that the ancestor is not a spirit, or zombie that randomly strikes an offending

descendant with an illness, but as a departed elder
(okpako ro kpori) whose moral authority even in death
is deployed to enforce moral behaviour among his/her
descendants.

Ancestor Spirit Anger Belief as Theory

Now we come to the question as to whether the ancestor
spirit anger belief can be treated as the equivalent of a
scientific theory. Scientific knowledge advances through
stepwise scrutiny of theory defined as an exposition of an
abstract principle, or speculation as opposed to practice.
The question is: What should we make of traditional
African beliefs which evolved, we have to assume, to
guide African societies, for thousands of years, in social
and moral cohesion? How did the beliefs come about?
Are they superstitious non-science and therefore
nonsense, as they have been usually portrayed in colonial
writings? Or, are traditional African beliefs the
equivalent of theories that have within them grains of
essential truths about life in the environments in which
the beliefs evolved?

Professor Robin Horton of the University of Port
Harcourt, a major thinker in the modern era, brings a
background of western science and philosophy, as well as
considerable exposure to Kalabari religion, to bear on a
serious attempt at understanding traditional African
thought in comparison to scientific theory. Although
some of his conclusions are controversial, his work as a
whole is nevertheless important because it challenges the
modern scientists on what to make of traditional African
religious beliefs. It is useful to briefly refer, at this stage,
to an aspect of Horton's work that is relevant to the
discussion in this book, namely, ancestor spirit anger
belief as explanation for the occurrence of illness.

Horton's general conclusion is that traditional African religious beliefs are rational in the context of African culture as are scientific theories in the West. Traditional African religious beliefs are, in some senses, like scientific theories. This is an important conclusion from his many years of inquiry into the subject; it upholds the inherent rationality of traditional African beliefs, in contrast to the ancient sociologists' ideas that rationality was not the key to understanding such beliefs referred to in the second paragraph of this chapter.

Horton's basic argument is this: to the extent that the beliefs offer 'cause and effect' explanations, the beliefs are like scientific theories. For example, the ancestor spirit anger belief offers explanation for the occurrence of serious illness (the illness is caused by angered ancestor spirits), just as parasites, viruses, bacteria, cancer etc are explanations for the occurrence of illness in modern medicine. To that extent, African religious beliefs can be said to have something in common with scientific theory. But scientists quite rightly insist that a belief like the ancestor spirit anger explanation of illness does not contain enough information with which to test its validity: there are no empirical methods with which the existence of ancestor spirits can be verified. Hence, following Popper's criteria of demarcation of scientific from metaphysical propositions, traditional African beliefs of this kind are metaphysical, rather than scientific propositions.

The controversy surrounding Horton's work arises partly from a comparison of traditional African religious beliefs (e.g., belief in ancestor spirit anger as the cause of illness and such like), which in his view are representative of African modes of thought, with western scientific theoretical thinking (e.g., atomic theory and such like), which he considers to be representative of Western mode of thought.

This comparison of two unlike entities (one obviously religious, the other arcane science) led Horton to the conclusion that the African mode of thought is a 'closed predicament' whereas the Western mode is 'open'. By this he meant that the traditional African thinker cannot conceive of alternative explanations to those offered by his orthodox beliefs, whereas in the West, people are accustomed to challenging existing scientific theories[30]

This conclusion has been criticized on various grounds. In the context of the discussion in this book, it is apt to note is that traditional African religious beliefs are religious beliefs; by definition, all religious beliefs are closed predicaments and they are accepted in faith and not on the basis of empirical evidence. This is true of traditional African religious beliefs as it is of beliefs in other religions.

It is important to repeat here the point already made that even traditional Africans, many of whom hold the sort of religious belief under discussion, do not function in their everyday lives as if under the influence of such beliefs. It is therefore inappropriate to posit, as the 'closed predicament' argument does, that traditional Africans are people with closed minds, and are not open to alternative points of view.

We must note another characteristic of traditional African beliefs here, which is that such beliefs are all encompassing; there is no separation into fragments such

30 R. Horton, African traditional thought and western science', in: Rationality, B. R. Wilson, editor (Blackwell, 1976) p. 131-171.

that one belief is religion, another science or medicine or philosophy or sculpture etc.

According to Braithwaite:[31]

> It is within the religious frame work that the entire (African) culture resides. In other words, starting from this religious focus, there is no separation between religion and philosophy, religion and society, religion and art. Religion is the kernel of the culture.

It is therefore not surprising that an African belief such as the belief in ancestor spirit anger as an explanation for the occurrence of serious illness can also have the attributes of a scientific theory as Horton eloquently demonstrated; such attributes include the ability of the theory to offer cause and effect explanations of a phenomenon, as well as predict the events to which the theory relates.

The African ancestor spirit anger belief has these attributes: for example, a life-threatening illness has occurred and after divination and other accepted procedures have been undertaken, all concerned agree that the explanation for the occurrence of the illness is the anger of the ancestors, due to a sin committed by the sick person. All those caring for the patient i.e., the close kinship relations, the patient, diviner and everyone else in the community, accept the diviner's revelation that the illness is caused by ancestor spirit anger; the participants are by upbringing, part of the same medical culture; They are believers who accept the diviner's

31 E.K. Braithwaite, The African presence in Caribbean literature. Daedalus Journal of the American Academy of Arts and Science, (Cambridge, Harvard University Press, 1974) p. 4.

pronouncement in faith.

To all intents and purposes, the above scenario is not very different from what happens in modern medicine, where a medical team of specialists would examine the technology-derived diagnosis of illness (laboratory test results, X-rays etc) and from there decide on the cause of illness. To that extent, ancestor spirit anger belief works like a scientific theory and at that level of comparison, Horton's conclusion that traditional African beliefs are like theories in science is helpful. Furthermore, the belief also has predictive attributes, like a scientific theory: the belief predicts that if a believer (an acculturated individual) should commit the sort of sin that angers the ancestors, the ancestors may strike the offender down with serious illness. The association of serious illness with a prior sin committed by the ill person is continuously reinforced by anecdotes in African traditional communities.

Analogically, the theory in modern medicine that malaria disease is caused by plasmodium parasites transmitted by anopheles mosquitoes, predicts that if you expose yourself to anopheles mosquito bites, you may be develop malaria.

Thus although no empirical connection was ever established between illness and ancestor spirit anger, historical experience of the potency of the belief and its acceptance by faith meant that no empirical proof was needed for its acceptance as a valid doctrine. Because of this predictive attribute (that sin against the ancestors will result in serious illness) this belief plays an important role in the control of moral behaviour in traditional Urhobo societies. To be healthy, persons must avoid the kind of abomination that might anger the ancestors. As

I argue later in the book in connection with the Yoruba magun taboo belief, the question as to whether ancestors actually zap their offending descendants with serious illness, is not of critical importance; rather the power of the belief to control moral conduct among believers lies in the belief itself.

Although the religious configuration of ancestor spirit anger belief hinders its acceptance by empirical science as theory, it should be noted that it enabled the belief to function as a moral law, as well as a rational basis for dealing with serious illness in traditional Urhobo societies. And, if the proposition in this book, that the belief can be understood as a shorthand reference for sustained emotional distress is valid, then the belief can be discussed as a scientific theory.

Are traditional African cultures closed predicaments?

Horton's 'open' and 'closed' predicament argument touches on fundamental aspects of African thought. It is partly on the basis of such description of traditional African patterns of thought that some Western-trained minds may look on traditional African theoretical thinking as superstition. The idea that African traditional cultures are a closed predicament may be mistaken by some to imply that the African mind is closed to argument and to new ideas; whereas in fact, Africans are among the most open-minded and adaptable people on earth. Witness the relative ease (compared to say Asians) with which Africans are converted to religious faiths away from their traditional religions.

The argument is that in traditional (African) cultures there is no developed awareness of alternatives to the established body of theoretical tenets; whereas, in scientifically oriented cultures (the West), such awareness is highly developed. Thus traditional African cultures are described as 'closed predica-ments' and scientifically oriented cultures are 'open'. The legendary Professor Edward Evans-Pritchard of Witchcraft, Oracles and Magic among the Azande fame had written of the Azande and their witchcraft beliefs in the same vein as follows

> Their intellectual ingenuity and experimental keenness are conditioned by patterns of ritual behaviour and mystical belief. Within the limits set by these patterns, they show great intelligence, but it cannot operate beyond these limits. ...they reason excellently in the idiom of their beliefs, but they cannot reason outside or against their beliefs because they have no other idiom in which to express their thoughts.[32]

The Azande are a Sudanese tribe among whom Sir Edward Evans-Pritchard lived and studied witchcraft belief in the 1930s. The Azande, like other traditional African people, are imbued with strong beliefs in witchcraft, which they see as offering explanations to many of life's perplexing experiences. My point is that the Azande see no alternatives to the explanations offered by witchcraft beliefs because these beliefs are religious in nature.

Witchcraft belief adherents accept the existence and potency of witchcraft by faith. To the extent that a person in possession of witchcraft is believed to have supernatural spiritual powers, witchcraft belief is a religious belief. It is in the nature of human beings that

---

32 E.E. Evans-Pritchard, Witchcraft, Oracles and Magic among the Azande (London: Oxford University Press, 1937) p. 338.

we accept religious dogmas by faith. It is because of faith, that no believer seeks alternative explanations to Christian doctrines such as the Resurrection, Trinity, the Virgin Birth, the coming of the Messiah, etc. The traditional African thinker does not challenge his own orthodox beliefs because those beliefs have significant religious components.

Let me repeat for emphasis that anchoring the ancestor spirit anger belief on a religious framework served two purposes: (i) it enabled the belief to be used as a doctrine (incest is a sin punishable by the ancestors) in the upbringing of individuals and (ii) it functioned as a moral law in society.

Karl Popper and traditional African beliefs

Traditional African beliefs of the type under discussion are metaphysical statements, according to Karl Popper, scientific propositions can be distinguished from metaphysical state-ments, i.e. "Statements consisting mainly of theoretical speculations about the supernatural and magic".

Popper wrote: "for all genuine scientific statements an empirical verification and . . . an empirical falsification must both be logically possible", empiricism being "the principle that only experience can devide about the truth or falsity of a factual statement."[33] He went on to say:

> We adopt as our criterion of demarcation (between science and metaphysics) the criterion of falsifiability. According to this criterion statements... convey information

---

[33] K.R. Popper, The Logic of Scientific Discovery (8th Impression) (London, Hutchinson, 1975), p. 312.

> about the empirical world...only if they can be
> systematically tested, that is to say, if they can
> be subjected...to tests which might result in
> their falsification.[34]

A statement is acceptable as a scientific proposition only if it contains enough information which would enable the proposition to be proved wrong (falsified); if any aspectl of the statement can be falsified by empirical means (e.g. by experimental data) then the hypothesis must be rejected as meaningless. This is a most profound insight into the nature of science; it is by rigorously subjecting propositions to falsification tests that we can expect to come close to scientific truth; in fact in Popper's sense there can be no scientific truth, only theories which are for the time being not falsified.

A statement, for example, that a given illness is due to the anger of offended ancestors is a metaphysical statement by Popper's definition because it involves speculations about the existence of ancestors spirits; there are no empirical methods for demonstrating the existence of such spirits or for showing a causal relationship between them and an illness. Beliefs like these that do not contain enough verifiable information which would enable them to be subjected to falsification tests are metaphysical statements and must be differentiated from scientific hypotheses.

On the other hand, a statement that malaria parasites in the body of a person is the explanation for the person's fever, has enough information to allow the theory to be tested: Both the fever and malaria parasites in the sufferer's blood can be determined empirically.

---

[34] Ibid.

This theory is in fact the basis for the treatment of malaria fever. An empirical approach to falsification of the theory would be to break the causal relationship between the feverish condition and the presence of parasites in the patient's body. If, for example, the fever could be shown to subside by acceptable methods, despite the presence of parasites in the patient's blood, this would constitute a falsification of the original hypothesis, and if reproduced, would lead to a rejection of the theory that plasmodium parasites invariably cause raised body temperature. In science, there are no 'truths' only 'hypotheses' that have not been successfully challenged.

Metaphysics and empirical science

However, Popper warned that the discovery of the principle that science and metaphysics can be distinguished from one another on the basis of certain criteria should not be taken to imply that metaphysical theories are meaningless. He wrote that, "from a historical point of view metaphysics can be seen to be the source from which the theories of empirical science spring".[35]

Morris also wrote that religion serves "to connect things with each other, to establish internal relations between them, to classify and systematize them ... The essential ideas of science are of religious origin".[36] In both religious and scientific thinking the mind is grappling with how to give expression to an imagined reality; in religion we imagine what the reality of the

[35] Ibid.

[36] Morris, p.137

supernatural world might be like and from the perceived manifestation of that world and divine inspiration we concretize perception into beliefs and, and where applicable, sacred scriptures.

In science, from experience and observations of natural manifestations we imagine what laws connect these manifesta-tions and from those observations scientists formulate theories or hypotheses regarding natural laws. Belief in TAM , though not empirically derived, are statements representing cumulative experience of illness and the imagined role of the supernatural in its occurrence. In the particular case of ancestor spirit anger belief, the fact that sin or abomination was seen as the trigger of ancestor spirit anger suggests, that serious illness was strongly associated with immorality in traditional African thought: in other words, ancestor spirit anger belief is a moral law.

The purpose of the ancestor spirit anger belief

Here we may pause to reflect on how the ancestor spirit anger belief could have come about. Are ancestor spirit anger belief -driven illnesses self-inflicted? Did the belief evolve to create emotional turbulence and hence illness in people for no other ulterior purpose, or was the belief necessary for the survival of the kinship group? I am inclined to speculate that ancestor spirit anger belief evolved with a purpose (if one can talk of a purpose in this connection) which was to control moral conduct in small-scale African kinship groups. We see that the belief rests on three essential elements: (a) immoral conduct, (b) the ability of the acculturated individual's conscience to provoke an emotional response, and (c) the incorruptible supernatural ancestors, whose anger triggers the illness.

The belief in the power of high-ranking ancestors (Erinvwin) to enforce moral laws is a core concept in Ughievwen traditional religion. As a religious concept can we not think of it as a divine revelation inspired by the peoples' close observations and experience of human nature? Throughout human history, the divine has revealed itself to different people at different times in their different environments; that is why, according to John Tavener,[37] it is a misconception to think that it is only through one revelation that God can be understood:

> We have to understand that there are other revelations of God, the revelation of Hinduism, the revelation of Buddhism, the revelation given to the prophet of Islam and the revelation of virgin nature (given) to the American Indians. We have so much to learn from all of them.

One can add to this list the revelations of physical nature and of the supernatural to ancient Africans in their tropical environment, from which we should seek understanding. In small kinship groups where the seeds of ancestor spirit anger belief were sown, the need for social cohesion (necessary for group survival) must have been paramount, compelling strict adherence to moral norms as a critical imperative for group harmony. In the absence of a central law enforcement authority, who could the people trust to be impartial custodians and enforcers of moral laws, but the spirits of high ranking ancestors who had attained eternity and divinity?

---

[37] J. Tavener, "Primordial depth", in: BBC Belief, Jane Blakewell, editor, (Duckworth Overlook, London, 2005).

The idea that the ancestors could function as moral law-enforcing agents, could conceivably have evolved in such a milieu. I use the word 'evolved' deliberately. The forms in which the belief in ancestors is expressed in African societies today are most probably variants of its original form; changes have occurred with diversification in languages, dialects and cultures. This is evident from the common observation that although most peoples in sub-Saharan African subscribe to the belief in ancestors and their power to influence the fortunes of their living descendants, the mechanisms by which this influence is exerted varies greatly between African groups; as are the ways ancestors are acknowledged and celebrated. For example, as we shall see below in chapter 4, the Ughievwen venerate their ancestors through libation and elaborate festivals conducted annually in ways that are different in form from those of other Nigerian nationalities etc. These differences are not fundamental; they are different forms in which the logos of the ancestors and their influence in the lives of their descendants are celebrated and acknowledged. I am suggesting here that ancestor spirit anger belief evolved primarily as a mechanism for ensuring strict adherence to moral behaviour in traditional African kinship groups, but it does not follow that the association of immorality with serious illness in the acculturated individual is irrelevant in today's world.

Ancestor spirit anger explanation of illness as a metaphor

I have taken the belief to be a metaphor, a figure of speech, a symbolic shorthand statement encoding a more elaborate meaning which I interpret as sustained emotional distress. I arrived at this interpretation from direct observation of how the belief is used in actual situations of serious illness in Ughievwen society. The crystallization of experience into belief must have occurred over hundreds or thousands of years. The belief is so entrenched in the Ughievwen mindset, that it is difficult to convince the traditional thinker that the offended ancestors do not directly zap their victims with illness. This is despite the strong evidence from what they do in practice (see the next chapter), that the people must know that the cause of serious chronic life-threatening illness in an offending descendant is in his consciousness. When divination diagnosis points to emuerinvwin as the cause of illness the first thing the community of caregivers does is approach the ill person for a confession, for a confirmation, of the abomination. Confession and confirmation of the sin must happen before ritual sacrifices are made to appease the angered ancestor. This is a crucial step in the therapeutic procedure, which means that the people know that the origin of the illness is in the consciousness of the victim. Ancestor spirit anger is thus a metaphor.

This interpretation enables us to examine the belief from two perspectives: as a basis for understanding what hitherto appeared as obscure inexplicable procedures such as divination, incantations, sacrifices, unusual methods of application of plant remedies, etc, in TAM, particularly in the treatment of serious illness. These procedures are often mistakenly viewed in modern medicine circles as superstitious practices by ignorant people. My interpretation enables us to argue that these procedures are not mindless superstitions, but procedures that have the effect of diffusing mental stress and returning the patient to emotional equilibrium. Second, it brings the belief into the realm of a scientific proposition that can be evaluated in the context of current medical thinking, for example, in the context of research findings from psychoneuroimmunology.

Furthermore considering the time (probably thousands of years) that it must have taken fior traditional African experience of the relationship between anti-social conduct and illness, to crystallize into a belief, and the consistency that we see between the belief and TAM practices in African societies, it is fair to say that there is validity in this interpretation, on the basis of which the original idea can be treated as a scientific hypothesis and subjected to empirical verification. Understanding the belief as metaphor enables us to treat it as an overarching paradigm under which many of the activities of traditional healers take place, comparable to the germ theory of disease in modern medicine.

Science is not as open a culture as it is made out to be

From what has been said so far, it may appear that all scientific propositions are open to falsification, that there are no constraints on the activities of the scientist. However, it is common knowledge that the empirical scientists' choice of problems to research into are constrained by factors such as available facilities and methodology, current fashionable trends in the particular branch of science, access to funds, economic potential of the research findings etc. All these factors, individually or collectively compel the direction of scientific research. Therefore scientific activity is not always as open as one may infer from its characterization by Popper above. A scientist operates within a constraining theoretical framework, referred to by Thomas Kuhn as a paradigm "which is like an accepted judicial decision in the common law; it is an object for further articulation and specification under new or more stringent conditions".[38] A paradigm, like a Supreme Court judgement, is not overturned lightly. The majority of scientists work all their lives without questioning the overarching paradigm of their discipline: Medical research is constrined by the germ theory of disease, i.e., the overarching paradigm under which all activities of medical scientists, take place. In pharmacology the paradigm propelling drug discovery is selective toxicity i.e., the idea that for a chemical entity to be acceptable as a drug, it must show capacity to selectively poison the cause of disease. This means that most of the activities of the scientists in this field are focused on the search for specific receptor molecules that are relevant to a disease state, and chemical entities that have high affinity (agonists and antagonists) for those receptor molecules. Alternaive theories and debates usually go on for years concerning the mechanism of the killing action of a particular group of antibiotics or antiviral drugs, without a shift in the germ theory paradigm, which is that diseases are caused by germs, physical biochemical malfunctions, cancers etc whose removal with drugs or surgical excision will cure the disease.

Any explanation of illness that falls outside the ambit of the germ theory of disease is liable to be rejected as spurious by the community of pharmacologists. And, as Kuhn points out:

---

[38] T.S. Kuhn, The Structure of Scientific Revolution, 3rd ed, (Chicago, University of Chicago Press, 1996) p.23.

> One of the things a scientific community (of practitioners of a scientific specialty) acquires with a paradigm is a criterion for choosing problems. . . that can be assumed to have solutions. To a great extent these are the only problems that the community will admit as scientific or encourage its members to undertake. Other problems . . . are rejected as metaphysical. . . . A paradigm can for that matter, even insulate the community from socially important problems that are not reducible to the puzzle form, because they cannot be stated in terms of the conceptual and instrumental tools the paradigm supplies.[39]

Let us cast this in the context of our ongoing discussion. Theoretical African thoughts on disease causation such as the ancestor spirit anger belief cannot lead to formulations and technologies appropriate to the germ theory of disease: they cannot lead to formulations with immediate practical clinical applications, drug discovery or the Nobel Prize. It is for these reasons that the community of medical scientists do not consider TAM a serious subject for research.

A good example of how the leading authorities in a particular field of medical science can ensure that the status quo interest in the paradigm of the discipline is sustained, is the case of a brilliant physiologist (first class graduate) whose elevation to the full chair of physiology at the University of Ibadan was delayed because his research touched on aspects of traditional African medicine and his work was published in journals that

---

[39] Kuhn, p. 37.

were considered by his peers to be not mainstream physiology journals.

What constitutes a metaphysical, rather than a scientific proposition is not always clear cut; traditional African beliefs should not be dismissed offhand as superstitious non-science. In particular, beliefs relating to illness and its management merit conscious examination for scientific meaning because the beliefs embody knowledge of illness causation gained over centuries of experience and observation in the African environment.

The ancestor spirit anger explanation of illness is holistic
There is a sense in which the ancestor spirit anger explanation of illness is more 'open' than the germ theory of disease: in modern medicine, once the cause of a given illness has been identified (and this can be done even from a far-away laboratory) from exa`mination of a blood sample or other specimen, no other explanation outside the context of the causative agent can be entertained. If laboratory tests show that the illness is pneumonia confirmed by the presence of the relevant bacteria or virus, what else can anyone say? In African medicine on the other hand, the people including traditional healers, usually have no difficulty in accommodating the medical scientist's explanation, for example, that the illness is caused by identifiable pathogens or other body malfunctions. In my experience, what they would contend is that before the pathogen or cancer there was a prior emotional distress. People do not just get cancer! That a particular individual is afflicted is not the result of a mere statistical chance occurrence. Modern medicine is coming to the same kind of conclusion. Many cases of chronic illness

have been found to be associated with a prior history of emotional upheaval.

Why even try to interpret traditional African religious beliefs?

I have used the term "metaphor" throughout this discussion, simply as a reference to a figure of speech in which what is said has another meaning, roughly reminiscent of proverbs employed in African narratives. This is the sense in which my use of the term should be understood, as an aide memoir, not in the technical literary definition of metaphor.

"Proverbs are the palm oil with which words are eaten". This proverb is an example of a Nigerian saying with many layers of meaning. If you have eaten roasted or boiled yam or plantain with or without palm oil, you know the difference in the ease with which the morsel goes down the throat! If you are Urhobo and have enjoyed listening to ototas (spokesmen) wittily deploying proverbs in oratorical banter, then the proverb quoted above would not need an explanation or interpretation. You would recognize the imagery.

However, the ancestor spirit anger belief does not evoke obvious images of emotional distress; it simply says that if you do something to anger the ancestors they may, as a consequence, chastise you with illness; and there is no explicit suggestion from traditional healers that the belief is a metaphor. To that extent, it can be argued that the belief was not intended to be understood as a metaphor, proverb or parable with a deeper meaning, and that my interpretation of it as such is a forced one. Yet, from my observation of the way the belief is deployed in practice among the Ughievwen, and other evidence described below, this interpretation is inevitable.

I agonized about this until the cliché that there is nothing new under the sun became a truth! The issue of the interpretation of ritual symbols in African religious life has received attention in the anthropological literature. Briefly, we may take one strand of the arguments from the review by Professor Brian Morris in his book Anthropolgical Studies of Religion where he discusses the issue: One view is that we should not go gbeyond the enthnographic data and assign meanings to ritual symbols that are not evident or articulated by the people themselves as I have attempted to do with regard to the ancestor spirit anger belief.

The other view is that an interpretation of traditional beliefs is warranted, ie, that the opposite stand above is rather restrictive; that the task of the anthropologist is to uncover hidden meanings in ritual symbols.[40] Indeed, if we accept that traditional beleifs are rational concepts that historically guided the well-being of the African people in their particular environments; and if we are to learn from the experience that gave rise to those beliefs, it is imperative that we attempt to interpret and examine those beliefs for meaning, by closely observing how the beliefs are deployed in practice by contemporary healers, even if the people themselves do not articulate the beliefs in terms of ulterior meaning.

Two competing health care traditions in Africa

In Africa then, we have two health care traditions, each in its way, a closed predicament. Modern scientific

---

[40] Morris, p. 241.

medicine is a culture which can be considered a closed predicament, being constrained by the overarching germ theory of disease, which does not consider or permit an explanation of illness that falls outside its rubric; and traditional African medicine in which ancestor spirit anger belief as an explanation for the occurrence of illness is a constraining paradigm because its religious config-uration does not permit it to operate like a scientific theory.

These two health care traditions are, at best, not interacting beneficially, and at worst, they are mutually antagonistic. Yet both traditions have one goal--namely, to promote health care in Africa. The important practical question therefore is 'how can we bridge the two traditions, reconcile the contradictions, so that we can take the best ideas from each to advance human healthcare in Africa?

The future of health care for humanity lies in modern medicine, but because the ideas embedded in TAM beliefs are ecologically and culturally relevant to well-being in Africa, the beliefs ought to be scrutinized to know how modern medicine can benefit from them to improve the health of the African people. This is the main objective of this analysis.

Chapter 4

Evidence that Ancestor Spirit Anger Belief is a Metaphor

Ancestor spirit anger belief is a shorthand representation of the accumulated experience of sustained emotional distress arising from a hidden knowledge of antisocial conduct is the theory being tested in this chapter.

Support for this interpretation comes from two sources: One source is the observation of what traditional healers and their clients do, when faced with chronic serious illness, and the other is scientific evidence that emotional distress can be felt and that sustained negative emotions can predispose the individual experiencing the emotion to chronic illness.

Most of the information in the first category came from field observations and interviews with traditional healers in the Ughievwen communities of Delta State, Nigeria. Let us begin by considering upbringing. In traditional Ughievwen/ Urhobo society one is brought up to believe in the reality of the ancestors and their influence on the affairs of living descendants; it is a given that a violation of certain of society's moral laws would anger the ancestors who may knock down the offender with serious illness or death. This belief is strongly held and repeatedly reinforced by stories of serious illness or death caused by ancestors in the community. By this process of group acculturation, people grow up knowing that an emuerinvwin will draw the ire of the ancestors. Therefore, when an acculturated individual commits an abomination which he knows to be emuerinvwin, that person must respond with an autonomic upheaval, an attack of conscience, according to the model described by Professor Hans Eysenck in his famous book, Crime and Personality.[41]

In his model, conscience acts as deterrent against antisocial behaviour; the autonomic upheaval or attack of conscience experienced by an acculturated individual when contemplating an antisocial act is, for most people, strong enough to prevent the person from going through with his plan. But if the temptation over rides the 'voice' of conscience or the person's level of acculturation is not sufficient to hold him back from committing the act and he does, fear and anxiety over the possibility of ancestor spirit anger would persist and gnaw at him for as long as the abomination remains un-confessed resulting in emotional distress.

Eysenck points out the all too obvious fact that the majority of human beings are lawful members of society; the reason why this is so, why only a small proportion of human beings commit antisocial acts, is that the vast majority are sufficiently socialized to be deterred from criminal behaviour by an active conscience.

As suggested above, because the belief in ancestor spirit anger is a metaphysical/religious belief accepted in faith, it is used in the traditional upbringing of the young

---

[41] Hans Eysenck, (St Albans, Paladin Frogmore Press, 1977), p.114.

in traditional Urhobo society. What constitutes emuerinvwin, literally meaning "a matter on which only the ancestors can adjudicate" is common knowledge. The emotional response of an acculturated person to such a sin would be complex, consisting of anxiety and fear that the ancestors will, in due course, strike them with a serious illness or death. The other worries in the mind of such a person would include guilt, shame, and fear of loss of respect from disapproving kinship group members should the abomination come to light. These worries, sustained over time, combine to cause emotional distress.

My sense is that African ancients, over evolutionary time, came to the knowledge, through experience, that this state of mind can predispose the person undergoing the emotional distress to serious illness. The approximate Urhobo expression for emotional distress is ewen 'kpokpo hwo (the mind is troubling the person). Thus my interpretation of ancestor spirit anger as a metaphor for emotional distress would not surprise an Urhobo traditional thinker, if the point was stressed to him, although without conscious reflection, the typical traditional person would adopt a fundamentalist view that an angered ancestor, like a pathogen, directly inflicts illness on a transgressor.

Bodily response to emotions can be felt

To understand how the ancients, a preliterate people without formal knowledge of how the autonomic nervous system works, could have linked antisocial or immoral behaviour (emuerinv-win) to ill health, it may help to briefly reflect here on the biology of the human body's response to emotion: the physical body does respond to emotion in a way that can be felt by the person experiencing the emotion. It is most likely that the so called preliterate peoples' experience of such bodily response is at the heart of the evolution of the ancestor spirit anger belief.

In the following paragraphs, I describe the immediate response to emotions like fear, anxiety, hate, love/lust which are mediated by the autonomic nervous system, to demonstrate that the body's response to emotion can be felt; later in this section I expatiate more fully on the mechanisms, involving the endocrine, nervous and immune system pathways, that link negative emotions to illness; for which there is now empirical evidence from researches in the branch of medical science known as psychoneuroimmunology.

The human somatic response to emotion operates through the autonomic nervous system (ANS). The ANS is that part of the nervous system that functions independently of direct brain control. The ANS's manifestation in response to emotion is a well known fact of life employed in electronic devices called 'lie detectors'; these devices work on the principle that if a person consciously tells a lie to hide the truth which he knows, this contradiction provokes the autonomic nervous system of a socialized person to give out signals, for example, dramatic changes in heart rate, skin temperature, blood pressure etc, which the electronic devise can record. It is not just machines that can pick up these signals; people can experience their body's response when they try to hide the truth. Anyone going through the green Nothing to Declare customs gate at an airport, carrying what she/he knows, or suspects to be contraband

(Nigerians old enough to have lived through the eras of military dictatorships with their draconian laws, when one could not be sure whether one bottle of whiskey, wine or brandy bought at a duty-free shop in Europe, was a contraband in Lagos, or the person knew that the item was contraband, but tried to avoid declaring it (to avoid having to bribe the customs officer!) can testify to the body's anxiety response to this confusion. An experienced customs officer can pick out a potential offender by observing the 'body language' of the person who is trying to hide something!

Fear provokes a dramatic autonomic upheaval: if you have ever come face to face with a gun-wielding armed robber (as I have), you may recall that your heart was beating so furiously that you thought it would jump out of your chest! On the other hand, if you cast your mind back to when you unexpectedly came across your arch enemy on the corridors of your faculty, someone you really disliked, you may recall how strongly your body recoiled from the encounter. What if the person you unexpectedly came face to face with on the corridor was your lover? So, whether the human emotion is anxiety, fear, hate, love/lust, etc, the body autonomously responds in preparation for what may follow, in a way that can be felt by the person or that can be recorded electronically.

The ANS response to emotion is mediated by chemical substances released by autonomic nerves and/or endocrine glands; the actions of these chemical substances are widespread and may be cumulative, and if the emotion is negative, e.g., fear, hate, anger, envy etc, and is sustained, these chemical mediators can create conditions that are optimal for the occurrence of serious illness (also see stress below).

My speculation is that pre-literate man, over evolutionary time deduced the association between an immoral act and serious illness through the experience of bodily response to emotion.

Indications from TAM practice

Perhaps the most compelling ground for concluding that the ancestor spirit anger belief is a metaphor for emotional distress comes from observing the steps taken by care givers, that is, the ill person, his relatives, diviner and the elders of the kinship group, to ensure recovery when one of their members falls seriously ill. What suggests very strongly that ancestor spirit anger belief is a metaphor is that the people seem to know that the seat of serious illness is in the mind of the sufferer.

The following scenario enacted frequently among the Ughievwen community is characteristic of procedures taken when someone is struck down by serious life-threatening illness. A diviner (obo epha) is consulted for the purpose of determining the underlying spiritual cause of the illness. Usually by the time the illness is serious enough to compel divination (epha) consultation, and incur the expenses and the trouble of such consultation, those embarking on the consultation would already suspect that there is an underlying supernatural underpinning to the illness! The diviner, more often than not confirms the suspicion of the kinship group, for example, that the illness has its roots in ancestor spirit anger, in an emuerinvwin committed by the ill person. In many instances, the obo-epha does no more than hint at this possibility.

What the relatives of the sick person do on receiving such pronouncement is revealing; despite knowing who the offended ancestors must surely be in the particular case, no steps are taken to appease them (the ancestors) directly with ritual libation and sacrifices, which is what one would expect, if the people thought the angered ancestor, like a virus, was the direct cause of the illness and that the ill person was a passive victim of ancestor anger. Rather, those who consulted the diviner must first seek confirmation from the sick person. They will say to the ill person "we have consulted an obo-epha, from there we learned that this illness must be due to a serious wrongdoing, an emuerinvwin. Do you have any hidden sin?"

It is from the afflicted person's confession that he/she had indeed committed an emuerinvwin that the details of the abomination are brought to light. This must happen before the necessary ritual sacrifices are offered to the ancestors, asking them to forgive the offender. Characteristically, news of such confessions of emuerinvwin is 'eagerly and quickly broadcast' in the kinship community. That is how the moral law is propagated.

A confession of emuerinvwin is not difficult to obtain in these circumstances where a confession may mean the difference between life and death; also the sick individual having been acculturated and socialised in this culture, would have, during the course of a protracted illness, already been reflecting on the likely role of Erinvwin in relation to any hidden abomination, in his/her present predicament. An acculturated individual who committed incest, for example, would know from the moment the act was done, that he was in danger of ancestor spirit sanction with serious illness. He too would not be surprised at the diviner's pronouncement.

Another scenario is where an individual having committed an emuerinvwin in secret, subsequently finds the attack of conscience, fear of ancestor punishment gnawing at his consciousness unbearable, and he is forced to voluntarily confess the misdemeanour before the elders of the kinship lineage, to forestall ancestor spirit anger-induced serious illness. This is evidence that the acculturated individual in traditional African society may be under emotional stress from fear of ancestor spirit anger, if they have committed a grievous antisocial act. The different ways that ancestor spirit anger and serious illness are associated corresponding to the scenarios above, are illustrated by the actual cases I witnessed or that were reported to me in Ughievwen.

Case 1

A pregnant woman about 25 years, who we shall refer to as **MI**, had a difficult life-threatening labour during which she was moved from one maternity clinic to another in the town of Ijebu-Ode, where she and her husband were migrant labourers. Fearing the worst, close friends and relatives consulted an obo-epha (diviner) in the Urhobo enclave in the town; the diviner pronounced what everyone already suspected, namely, that **MI** had a secret which she must confess. When the lady failed to open up, she was taken on the four hour journey to her home village near Warri where, under pressure from her mother, she admitted that the pregnancy had occurred following intercourse with a lover before the marriage with her present husband was consummated; the pregnancy did not belong to her husband! After her confession she gave birth to a baby boy. Everyone agreed that her difficulty had been caused by ancestor spirit anger. This, described as a case of emuerinvwin, was narrated to me in 1980 by an eyewitness.

Case 2

I personally witnessed some aspects of this case in 1990. A man I shall refer to as AA, about 70 years old, took ill with what was eventually diagnosed at the general hospital at Ughelli (Ughelli North LGA of Delta State), as congestive heart failure. He was admitted, treated and later discharged with prescriptions for digoxin, diuretic and potassium supplement. Sadly, AA died at home shortly after he was discharged most probably, from my modern medicine perspective, because he did not continue to take his drugs. While he was still under hospital care, his two middle-aged daughters from a previous marriage had consulted a diviner to discover a possible spiritual cause of the illness. Congestive heart failure, of which the symptoms include swollen extremities, is an illness which the Ughievwen believe is likely caused by the supernatural for moral transgression. The diviner made the enigmatic pronouncement that their father's illness was something that he brought on himself. The diviner's pronouncement was made clear after AA's death. It transpired that two years earlier, AA's current wife and a neighbour had a dispute and had sworn before a highly feared local deity to use its powers to punish the guilty party in the dispute. AA, not wanting any harm to come to his young wife and their young children, had performed other rituals in an attempt to deflect the local deity's punishment away from her, should it happen that she was guilty, or possibly, knowing that she was guilty. The diviner's pronouncement was now interpreted to mean that AA's illness and subsequent death came about because he had attempted to interfere with supernatural justice. The facts had been revealed after AA's death; the daughters blamed their stepmother who they suspected knew of their father's abomination but did not tell what she knew. To prevent the deity's further harm to AA's family, the whole conflict had to be resolved in the open before AA's final funeral rites. The deity's curse would have to be publicly revoked by its high priests. Meanwhile, libations and prayers were offered to reconcile the daughters and their stepmother. All the procedures including a full statement of the facts took place in public in the presence of the kinship group including this writer, during AA's final funeral ceremonies.

These two cases show that although certain difficulties (difficult child birth in case 1 and a serious illness in case 2), were attributed to punishment from angered ancestors or deity, the people understood, in practice, that whatever the problem was, it had to do with awareness of a misdemeanour in the consciousness of the sufferer.

Case 3

This case came to my attention in Owahwa in 1996. It concerns a former civil servant employee, BB, who had been forced out of his job because he had become physically handicapped. He now lived in the village with his large family with neither salary nor pension benefits.

He complained bitterly and wrote numerous petitions soliciting for his retirement benefits to be paid, to no avail. Over the years his health gradually deteriorated and despite the attention of local traditional healers his health did not improve. His condition was dire. Eventually, he told the oldest man in his immediate lineage, and later also the wider kinship group about his worries. He feared that his problems —his physical handicap, retirement with no benefits and his illness—may all be punishment for what in hindsight might have been an emuerinvwin. In the distant past, he had accidently seen his brother's wife naked. Although no intercourse had taken place beyond that, he was concerned, and obviously had wondered for some time, whether he was being punished for being in a position to see his brother's wife and therefore felt guilty of having sex with the woman vicariously. It was possible that the idea of sexual intercourse crossed his mind fleetingly at the time, which would be a grievous abomination in Urhobo moral law! Even though libations and relevant sacrifices were made to Erinvwin, BB eventually died of his illness. Members of the kinship group concluded that Erinvwin killed him.

I discussed this case with some elders. Why would Erinvwin kill the man after he had confessed his fears and libations and the relevant sacrifices had been offered to the ancestors? The view was that he died because his confession, now being interpreted as having had sexual intercourse with his brother's wife, could not be forgiven by Erinvwin. What then is the point of a confession if despite it, Erinvwin would kill?

My understanding is that in the management of a life-threatening illness in TAM, an attempt is made to restore the sick person to emotional equilibrium. This is achieved partly by confessions of emuerinvwin committed in secret, but the preservation of the power of the ancestors to continue to protect the society's moral integrity seems to be just as important a consideration. The death of BB, who seemed to have angered the ancestors, would have been understood in this context.

Case 4

In this case a man who shall be referred to as ED aged about 60—fearing that his apparent impotence might drive his young attractive wife into sexual intercourse with another man in search of more children—arranged with his younger cousin to have intercourse with her; if she became pregnant he hoped no one would know the truth. After some time had elapsed, it began to dawn on ED that what he had done was emuerinvwin and it would be a matter of time before Erinvwin struck him down with a serious illness. He panicked and summoned a meeting of the elders of the kinship lineage before whom he confessed his misdemeanour. ED and his younger cousin were fined and appropriate ritual sacrifices made to propitiate Erinvwin. ED and his cousin were thus saved, but when the cousin's daughter from his legitimate wife died later, the death was blamed on Erinvwin.

These two cases demonstrate that knowledge of an immoral act, an emuerinvwin, committed by an acculturated individual remains in the consciousness of the person, worrying him/her, long after the abomination. My contention is that traditional African societies knew this from experience and linked it to the occurrence of serious illness. Over a period of many centuries this experience evolved into a mnemonic metaphor as belief.

The belief in Erinvwin, or the spirits of dead ancestors in general, and their ability to sanction descendants for immoral conduct is widespread worldwide. Margaret Mead[42] reported the following case in Papua New Guinea which prompted her to remark that "obligation to confess sins is accompanied by obligation to confess sins accidentally witnessed". Ten-year old Paleao had accidentally come upon his 35-year old cousin copulating with the 50-year old wife of his (the cousin's) uncle. He was shocked by what he saw, but he was old enough to know that this was a grievous sin against the ancestors. Sure enough the cousin became seriously ill with cerebral malaria some time after the incident, and lay in a coma. Paleao bravely rose to the occasion and described what he saw in order to save his cousin's life. Later, Paleao would say of his cousin "He would surely have died, and as a spirit, angry over his death, he would have killed me who had known the truth and concealed it".

Thus we can conclude that believers in the ancestor spirit anger explanation of illness recognize, though they do not so explicitly state it, that in life-threatening illness which they ascribe to emuerinvwin, the cause of the problem is in the mind of the sick person, who must first publicly acknowledge the sinful act, thereby purging himself of the burden of guilt.

---

[42] M. Mead, Growing Up in New Guinea. (London, Penguin Books, 1942) p. 129.

An individual socialized from childhood to know the type of antisocial behaviour that constitutes emuerinvwin, also knows the health significance of committing it. Therefore, the sinner would live with the knowledge of the guilt from the moment the abomination was committed, and from then on, every time he/she came in contact with those connected with or affected by the misdemeanour which, in the case of incest in close-knit, small kinship communities, would be often.

The scientific evidence is that sustained suffering from the complex of negative emotions arising from an antisocial act in a socialized individual would have the effect of lowering the person's immune capacity, and so making that individual more susceptible to illness than a person with a clean conscience. As has been said already, an adult Urhobo, when pushed to think about it, would accept that sustained emotional distress (ewen kpo kpo hwo, i.e., a troubled mind) can cause illness, but he would not want to take ancestor spirit anger out of the equation in particular cases of serious illness. He would argue, correctly according to my interpretation, that the troubled mind arose from fear/anxiety about ancestor spirit anger.

Evidence from Science

We now turn to what science has to say about the relationship between sustained emotional distress and the occurrence of serious illness. Can sustained emotional disequilibrium cause chronic life-threatening illnesses? What is being suggested is that an acculturated individual living with the knowledge of emuerinvwin, would experience a sustained attack of conscience which could render him susceptible to serious illness. Is there scientific evidence for this? The concept of emotional stress as a risk factor chronic illness in modern medicine is, in effect, similar to the concept of emuerinvwin in traditional Urhobo thought.

Stress

According to Hans Selye to whom the discovery of the concept of stress is credited, stress is the non-specific response of the body to any stimuli that upset the body's steady state equilibrium.[43] Factors that can cause stress include infections of any kind, disease, starvation etc; if we add upset of the steady state equilibrium of the external milieu, then other risk factors would include excessive physical exertion

Hans Selye's description of his first encounter with seriously ill patients as a medical student is worth recalling because it closely reflects the way Africans in traditional society, without diagnostic technology, see an ill person; as someone in whom the steady state equilibrium is disturbed. Selye tells us that what struck him on seeing the clinical cases of seriously ill patients presented by his professor of medicine was the similarity in their appearance. The patients all looked ill; they were emaciated, pale, weak and miserable. It did not matter whether the cause of illness was infection by staphylococcus, pneumo-coccus or tuberculosis, a virus or cancer, the patients presented generally miserable

---

[43] H. Selye, The Stress of Life, (New York: McGraw-Hill, 1978) p.12.

appearances that were indistinguishable until the specific cause of the illness was revealed by detailed scientific diagnosis.

Selye was to reach the profound conclusion years later that being ill was not the direct result of the infection or the cancer, but the result of the body's reaction to the infection, in an attempt to contain it. He referred to the body's reaction to the presence of the infective agent as a nonspecific adaptation syndrome. In this view it is the body's fight to control, and adapt to the presence of the pathogenic agent that constitutes illness; without it there is no illness. So, what we are saying is that the traditional African healer perceives in a seriously ill person the manifestation of a nonspecific adaptation syndrome, not a specific disease whatever it may be.

Selye's classical experiments showed that when laboratory animals are subjected to sustained stress (physical and emotional), the adrenal glands become enlarged, the stomach becomes ulcerated, the production of adrenaline (which increases blood pressure and blood sugar) and corticosteroids (which reduce resistance to infection) is increased; whereas functions of the immune system that protect the animal against infections are suppressed.

The general picture is the same in the human. People are more prone to illness when under stress (physical and emotional) than when they are not. What we are saying apropos ancestor anger belief is that an acculturated individual who commits a moral transgression is under emotional stress and, if sustained, can become more susceptible to serious illness than a person with a clean conscience.

The concept of emuerinvwin has universal health relevance

The idea that antisocial or immoral behaviour is bad for one's health, which is embodied in the Urhobo concept of emuerinvwin has resonance in current thinking in modern medicine where chronic serious illnesses are increasingly being associated with prior experience of emotional upheaval. The list of items recognized as stressors (that is, risk factors for serious illness) in the medical literature is long, but prominent among them is sustained emotional distress.

In general emotional distress may arise from any unfortunate life experience such as a painful separation from a loved one, bereavement, divorce and other emotional and physical trauma. Life styles and personality types that predispose individuals to certain kinds of stress have been identified and classified according to diseases such as heart attack or diabetes with which the personality type is associated.

People who spend their lives acting rudely and aggressively to those around them will alienate everyone in time; and the lack of social contact is known to be associated with a whole range of different illnesses. The reverse behaviours of love and compassion, kindness, moral integrity etc, are conducive to good health.

A famous Urhobo singer/songwriter "Professor" Aja, makes the following telling comment in his popular song

'Agha' (what we forbid) in which he urges his compatriots to abide by the traditions of their forebears. He sings:

'Ne Erinvwin re township nyo oyibo o, jo nyo yibo!

They think Erinvwin in the township does not hear English, but it hears English!

This is a warning to any Urhobo person living in urban areas, in the diaspora, not to think that because they are far away from their ancestral homes and now speak to one another in English, they can do what is forbidden and Erinvwin would not know!

Evidence that emotional experience affects a person's immunity

Negative emotions such as fear, guilt, anger, sustained anxiety, hate, feelings of insecurity, bereavement and boredom, borne over a period of time, are known stressors.[44] Although it has been known for long that emotional distress can manifest in physical ill health (psychosomatic medicine), it is only recently that the neural pathways linking emotion and somatic manifestations of illness have become reasonably well defined. Psychosomatic medicine tried to establish a correlation between psychosocial and biological factors in health and disease and in the process revealed that what are now referred to as autoimmune diseases —rheumatoid arthritis, systemic lupus erythematosus, multiple sclerosis,

---

[44] R. Charles, Mind, Body and Immunity, How to enhance your body's natural defences (London, Methuen, 1990) p. 99-103.

ulcerative colitis etc.,—are underpinned by psychosocial factors.

But psychosomatic medicine failed to identify the part played by the immune system in the interaction between mind and body to cause disease. In fact it failed to stem the drift towards the dichotomy between mind and body that modern medicine brought about, by its advances in diagnostic technology and molecular biology which led increasingly to the notion that one could know all about an illness by scientific examination of disease specimens or biopsy, and by the use of powerful selectively acting drugs.

Research findings in the last three decades in the sub-speciality called psychoneuroimmunology (PNI) are now opening up the mechanistic pathways linking the nervous, endocrine and the immune systems to emotional experience that can impact on health. PNI has been described as "a singular field . . . with roots in holistic practices of traditional medicine".[45]

Here are some facts in the story of how science came to the conclusion that the brain controls immunity, which is the central idea in psychoneuroimmunology: In 1984 adreno-corticotrophic hormone (ACTH) was shown to occur in lymphocytes;[46] ACTH is a hormone hitherto thought to be made only in the anterior pituitary region of

[45] M.L. Lyon, Order and healing: The concept of order and its importance in the conceptualisation of healing. *Medical Anthro-pology,* 1990 (12): 249 - 268.

[46] J.C. Blalock, Shared ligands and receptors as a molecular mechanism of communication between the immune and neuro-endocrine systems, Annals of the New York Academy of Science, 1994, 741, 292-298.

the brain. The occurrence of this substance in immune cells (lymphocytes) in circulating blood was a clue that communication between the immune system and the brain is a two-way affair. Blalock and colleagues concluded from extensive research in this area that the "cells of the immune system might function in a sensory capacity, signalling to the neuro-endocrine system in response to non-cognitive stimuli" such as viral or bacterial infections via peptides common to both immune and neuro-endocrine systems. White blood cells (lymphocytes) can produce lymphokines to which the nervous system responds and the functions of these lymphocytes are affected by the messages they receive from the brain, thereby acting like bits of the brain in circulation.

In response to an emotional experience, the brain releases chemical mediators which react with immune cells in circulation, with a consequent change in the immune status of the person experiencing the emotion. Cells of the immune system can respond to the autonomic nervous system (ANS) neurotransmitters or hormones released from the brain when a person is under emotional stress; lymphocytes possess receptors for many central nervous system and ANS neurotransmitters. Furthermore, immune organs such as the spleen have dense sympathetic nerve supplies with evidence of complicated "cross talk' between spleen cells and sympathetic neurotransmitters.[47]

What I have described above is a very brief sketch from a massive body of data showing that the brain

---

[47] H.R. Straub, Complexity of the bi-directional neuro-immune junction in the spleen, Trends in Pharmacological Sciences 2004 (25): 640-646.

controls immunity in a person by virtue of the emotions experienced by that person. Negative emotions of fear, hatred, envy, anger, anxiety, sense of loss etc, are known to lower the immunity of a person experiencing the emotion, whereas the opposite emotions of love, compassion, happiness etc may stabilize the immune status. The traditional African experience that gave rise to the ancestor spirit anger theory under discussion is consistent with the science: If an acculturated individual commits an antisocial act (emuerinvwin) he will be under such sustained emotional distress as to depress the individual's immune system, thereby making the person to be more susceptible to illness than a person who is not under such emotional stress.

The role of ancestor spirit anger belief in the control of behaviour

If, as pointed out earlier, the people in traditional African societies knew from experience that a "troubled mind" (ewen kpo kpo hwo) can predispose one to serious illness and that confessions of sin are critically important steps in the management of serious illness, then why is the idea embedded in a religious construct, in a belief that attributes serious illness to the anger of dead ancestors? Why do they not simply say that the illness is due to a "troubled mind"? I suggest that the religious configuration of the belief serves at least two purposes (if one can be permitted to speak of 'purpose' in the context of belief):

    i.   it served as a shorthand explanation for the occurrence of serious life-threatening illness

whose specific cause could not be otherwise
ascertained

ii. It served as a moral law—the fear of serious illness
and possibly death due to ancestor spirit
anger—deterred people from antisocial behaviour
of the type that were recognized as punishable by
the ancestors (emuerinv-win).

It made people to live within society's critical moral laws,
especially those related to incest, which posed serious
threat to group harmony and social cohesion.

We may pause here to reflect on why adherence to
moral law might have been of paramount importance in
early human societies. In the absence of centralized law
enforcement authorities such as law courts and the police,
strict adherence to societies' moral laws was the
mechanism by which society ensured harmony and
cohesion among its members. Urhobo society did not
have indigenous centralized law enforcement agencies
before colonial governments introduced them. Until then,
governance was based on gerontocracy and benevolent
theocracy in autonomous village or town republics. It was
therefore important for such societies to inculcate in their
members the society's critical moral norms, by the most
effective means possible. Because the ancestor spirit
anger belief was constructed as a religious dogma and
accepted in faith, it could be incorporated into
socialization schemes in the upbringing of the individual.

We have speculated above that the instinct that drove
the evolution of the ancestor spirit anger belief was group
survival, and the imperative for adherence to strict moral

conduct. Ancestor spirit anger belief became an effective mechanism for, among other functions, mobilization of kinship group members against potentially self-destructive antisocial behaviour.

Divination and confession

If we now examine the methods used by TAM practitioners to intervene in serious illness we see that diffusion of emotional tension is indeed a major therapeutic objective. Divination is the diagnostic procedure that reveals supernatural underpin-nings of illness. Divination is defined in greater detail in the next chapter; here I simply want to stress that the role of the diviner is critically important in illness management in African medicine. It is the diviner who, having pointed to a supernatural agency as the likely cause of an illness is the initiator of confessions by the sick person. This procedure has at least two effects: one is the diffusion of emotional tension. For the first time since committing an emuerinvwin, the sick person has the opportunity, albeit under pressure, to narrate publicly the details of the guilt that has for long gnawed at his consciousness. This must represent liberation from emotional stress for the individual and for the kinship group whose members might have been directly or indirectly affected by the sick person's misdemeanour.

Second, the diviner plays a crucial role in the continuation and affirmation of ancestor spirit anger belief. Confessions of antisocial act quickly become public knowledge among members of the kinship group and even in the wider community. This means that the community's moral norms and the consequences of their breach are repeatedly and vividly made known in the community. Confessions have the effect of diffusing emotional tension in the kinship group and may help to restore the sick person to health through a surge in immune activity.

The idea of personal guilt resulting in illness attributed to the anger of the ancestors or a deity seems to have been with humanity at different times and places, and calls to mind this segment of a classic Christian prayer:

> O Heavenly Father, who in thy Son Jesus Christ, has given us a true faith, and a sure hope; help us, we pray thee, to live as those who believe and trust in the communion of saints, the forgiveness of sins and the resurrection of life everlasting. Strengthen this faith and hope in all the days of our lives [my italics for emphasis].

The treatment was successful but the patient died
It can be seen that the success or failure of treatment of serious illness in TAM is not to be judged solely by whether the sick person was cured of the illness or not. The procedures adopted serve wider social purposes in addition to the immediate objective of healing the ill person. A reaffirmation of the moral norms of the community and its stand against antisocial behaviour is one important purpose. Treatment of illness in TAM is thus holistic in a very broad sense —the treatment may

heal the person but it may also heal the kinship group. As Kleinman [48] says in connection with traditional healing practices in general,

> . . . healing is evaluated as successful (when) the sickness and its treatment have received meaningful explanations (and). . . related social tensions and threatened cultural principles have been dealt with appropriately.

There is indeed a sense in which we can say that in traditional African culture, the reaffirmation of society's moral norms for which serious illness of a transgressor provides an opportunity, is at least as important an objective as the restoration of health to the transgressor. As has been suggested above, the ancestor spirit anger belief probably evolved with the main purpose to ensure moral conduct among early human populations. If serious illness occurred and this was because, according to belief, the ill person had committed what is considered an immorality capable of triggering ancestor spirit anger, this would be proof that the ancestors were effectively in control of moral behaviour among the descendants. If despite all appropriate processes, the patient still died, that death might be viewed positively as evidence that the belief system was effective in controlling moral conduct (how could a person who committed such a heinous sin live, if indeed the

---

[48] A. Kleinman, Concepts and a model for the comparison of medical systems as cultural systems. in: Concepts of Health, Illness and Disease Caroline Currer and Margaret Stacey, editors (Oxford, Bergamon Press, 1993).

ancestors were alive to their responsibilities!). And, the death of the sinner may be viewed as a warning to other members of the kinship group against such an antisocial behaviour.

This seems to be the general attitude of the community to the death of someone who had confessed to an emurinvwin. In Case 3 cited above, for example, what members of the kinship group, i.e., brothers, uncles, nephews, cousins etc, most frequently referred to after the death of BB, was the fact that he had committed a terrible abomination, more than the fact that his death was a serious loss to his immediate family, the kinship lineage and community at large. It was as if the consolidation of the group's moral integrity was more important than the loss of their member who had committed an emuerinvwin. It meant that such a person had forfeited the right to live in the community.

PART TWO

Organization of TAM Practices
and the Concepts and the Instruments Deployed
in the Management of Serious Illness

In African medicine, there are no laid down procedures is followed by practitioners; in general, there is very little interaction between different healers and there are no formalized mechanisms for the exchange of ideas on professional practice as we have in modern medicine, where such exchanges take place regularly in medical books, scientific publications and in the electronic media. Furthermore, in African medicine, there is no agreement on what conditions one has to fulfill in order to be accepted and inducted into the traditional healing profession, unlike what obtains in modern medicine.

Despite this apparent absence of lines of communication between practitioners, certain concepts and instruments that are unique to TAM practice can be identified. Thus, although TAM can be said to be characterized by informality and improvisation, complex beliefs such as divination, incantation, witchcraft, the curse etc, that are important features of TAM practice and deployed in the management of serious illness, have survived. These ideas are further defined and discussed in this part of the book. Their analyses reveal that these practices and beliefs, like the ancestor spirit anger belief, are a reflection of the strong association between antisocial/immoral conduct and serious illness in the traditional African thought.

Chapter 5

Induction into the Healing Profession in African Medicine

<hr>

C laims that long periods of formal training or apprenticeship are required before one can be recognized as a traditional healer abound (e.g., up to 15 years).[49] Una Maclean's well-known study of traditional healers in the semi-urban metropolis of Ibadan, Nigeria—where the practice of traditional African medicine (TAM) even 40 years ago, was already acquiring the characteristics of modern business requiring many different competencies. While there can be no argument that some degree of exposure (training/ apprenticeship) in a traditional medicine environment must be necessary for individuals to become healers, the insistence by articulate urban herbalists that such exposure was a formal and routine requirement, is reminiscent of other claims made by urban "professional" healers to enhance their image, to give the impression that their qualifications are comparable to

<hr>

[49] Una Maclean, Choices of Treatment among the Yoruba, in: Culture and Curing, Perspectives on traditional medical beliefs and practices P. Morley and R. Willis, editors, (London: Peter Owen Ltd, 1978) p. 163.

what obtains in modern medicine. In the latter, a long period of formal training of personnel (doctors up to 7 years, pharmacists and others up to 5 or 6 years to obtain a basic qualification) is an accepted prerequisite for induction into the profession.

My impression from observations in rural Ughievwen is that people come into the practice of TAM by routes other than formal training or apprenticeship. The modes of recruitment which I identified are similar to the general mode of induction into the role of inganga (healer) among the BaKongo of the lower Zaire described by Jansen.[50] The following modes based on Jansen's outline are probably representative of, and applicable to, modes of induction into TAM practice in many parts of Africa.

Modes of Induction into TAM

i. Having a visionary encounter with the spirit world during a personal trauma or illness

One of the subjects I interviewed in this study, Saradje (not his real name) stated that while he lay awake at night worrying about his illness (he had been told he had severe hypertension, but could not afford the drugs), he saw in his mind's eye, as it were, that the bark of the tree

---

[50] J.M. Janzen, The Quest for Therapy: Medical pluralism in the Lower Zaire, (Berkeley: University of California Press, 1978) p. 196.

Newbouldia laevis[51] (Oghriki in Urhobo) would cure him. On the basis of this revelation, he removed oghriki bark, dried it in the sun, pounded it a little, macerated it in a local gin (ogogoro) and began taking a small quantity of the decoction daily until he became well again and, as he put it, his young wife became much happier with him; even though he had had no prior experience of oghriki's efficacy, nor had he been a traditional healer of any note up to that point (he was in fact a well known tailor in the community). From then on Saraje said he recommended oghriki bark to others who were ill with similar symptoms. This is characteristic of how the informal system operated: Overtime Saradje acquired a reputation as a traditional healer in Owahwa.

Barbara Lex[52] suggests that in traditional medicine, apprenticeship can be acquired through personal illness, resulting in a heightened ability to recognize the possible cures that are available in nature.

ii. Being an apprentice to a master healer purchasing treatments, for example, an apprentice may assume the role purchasing treatments, (sourcing the herbs) and experimenting with individual cures.

---

51 Newbouldia laevis is a well-known tree in Nigeria. The Urhobo use it as hedge to mark off shrines and places of worship. It is also used as boundary marker; once the tree takes root, it is difficult to remove. It survives 'burn and slash' used to clear bush in preparation for planting; the tap root is large and buried deep in the soil. In Yorubaland the leaves are used in the ceremony of iwuye investiture of traditional chieftaincy.

52 Barbara Lex, Voodoo Death: New thoughts on an old explanation. American Anthropologist 76, (1974); 818-833.

iii. Induction into the profession through force of circumstances.

For example, a bonesetter may have fallen from a palm tree and broken a bone before seeking apprenticeship. A woman may have been obliged to purchase a remedy for a sick child and then using it to treat others as a favour. People in traditional society tend to pass on 'knowledge' of medicines based on personal experience, sometimes with dire consequences.

iv. A son or ward may imbibe the principles and practice of TAM from a practitioner parent or guardian

These informal modes of induction stand in sharp contrast to the practice in modern medicine where the doctor's training is a long process of professional indoctrination aimed at equipping the trainee with a body of scientific and specialist medical knowledge and skills that are largely unavailable to ordinary people. This gives the doctor a dominant authority in health matters such that the patient is often excluded from participating in crucial decisions in the management of his own illness.

The patient may be forced to become uncritically dependent on the pronouncements of the doctor and the medical profession as a whole. Ivan Illich[53] calls this the 'medicalization of life' whereby the medical profession

---

[53] Ivan Illich Medical Nemesis: The expropriation of health, (London: Calder and Boyers Ltd, 1975) p. 31.

has succeeded in taking away an individual's responsibility for his/her own well-being. It has reached the point where the medical profession now wishes to exercise professional control over what would have been regarded in traditional human life as normal events of life, e.g., pregnancy or growing old.

The traditional healer, whatever his mode of induction, is not the exclusive custodian of knowledge about health matters because as pointed out already the rules that govern wellness and illness in traditional African life are the same as those that govern moral and social harmonious relationships; individuals in traditional African societies were brought up to know, and they generally lived by, these rules.

Also, in general, the herbal remedies used in the treatment of minor ailments are usually common knowledge. In this respect African medicine is a way of life. No one had to be specially trained to understand the rules of behaviour that govern well-being. And, as already emphasized, in the event of a breach of the moral code and serious illness results, the facts of the antecedent antisocial conduct, and the rituals to placate the offended spirits and thus cleanse the system are performed in full view of the kinship public. The rules are thus repeatedly and publicly rehearsed.

It takes about seven years for a young person to acquire the basic knowledge to practice medicine; it will take another four for a clever doctor to go through residency to qualify as a specialist. The knowledge possessed by the modern doctor about disease is not common knowledge, it is vast, continuously expanding and completely outside the compass of his patients. Based on arcane scientific theories, the doctor can diagnose the cause of disease from a biopsy, blood or urine sample, and the patient does not have to participate in the process.

A word on the issue of secrecy in African medicine

People often say of African medicine practitioners that they are secretive and unwilling to share their knowledge with scientists. When the practitioner dies his knowledge dies with him; the death of an African wise man is like the loss of a library of rare books, is common cliché. This is largely true, but what is referred to as secrecy may also be a problem of communication common to word-of-mouth knowledge systems, and it is exacerbated when the communication is across cultural boundaries, for example, between an unlettered traditional healer and a western-trained medical scientist. The elite African medical scientist has to share part of the blame for the existence of this so-called secrecy.

The medical scientist who approaches the traditional healer as an interrogator, expecting the healer to discuss his methods in the scientific idioms of biomedicine is barking up the wrong tree. The traditional healer may not wish to explain why he makes certain incantations that he considers to be a necessary part of the treatment process; he may not explain why his medicines are not dispensed in precise doses.

In addition, the healer is all too aware that the medical scientist is coming from a background of what everyone agrees is superior Western technology and this is evident from the differences in material status between him and the healer: the medical scientist arrives at the mud hut abode of the healer in a motorcar, an embodiment of Western culture that has, for centuries, denigrated the healer's methods as irrational superstitions. That is not all, traditional healers quite rightly see themselves as custodians of an African cultural heritage and may be reluctant to give information that the scientist may go away and exploit, out of context, for financial gain. It is my experience, however, that even an unlettered traditional healer will talk freely about his work if he first gains the trust of the medical scientist in an atmosphere of mutual respect.

Let me conclude this chapter by reiterating that the accusation of secrecy levelled against traditional healers is partly a reaction on the part of the healers to the nonchalance of the educated medical practitioner who doubts whether there is anything to be gained from a serious scholarly engagement with practitioners of traditional medicine. In general, the African elite tend to see themselves as fortunate individuals who have been lifted above traditional institutions by Western education; especially during the years when they are in hot pursuit of career goals in the highly competitive field of modern medicine. There are few scholars of my generation in Nigeria (70 years and above) who would not admit that it has been in their later years that they came to the realization that traditional African institutions have something valuable to offer. This realization dawns gradually. After many years of seeing the world through the lens of European models which have not always been outstandingly successful in finding solutions to African problems, it is not surprising that educated Africans, who have worked these models all their lives should turn round to traditional institutions for another view of the world.

Chapter 6

Specialists in the Management of Serious Illness

T o stress the significance of the point I have made earlier that it is during the management of serious life-threatening illness that traditional religious consultations are made in African medicine, it is important to elaborate on the conceptual categorization of illnesses as 'major' or 'minor' in modern and African medicine. In what are usually referred to as minor ailments e.g., fever, aches and pains—the sufferer knows or can find out from a neighbour or family member roughly what the matter is and what to do about it, and would apply an appropriate treatment; that is to say, the ailment is self-diagnosed and self-medicated, without the doctor's prescription or without recourse to esoteric consultations. Then there is what I have referred to several times as serious life-threatening illness, in which a resolution requires the attention of a specialist.

Minor and serious illness can be a continuum. What may appear to be a minor discomfort may be the symptom or an early stage of a major life-threatening illness, e.g. a headache may be the symptom of an underlying life-threatening hypertension or brain tumour. Hence the usual warning in modern medicine following a completion of the recommended dose of e.g., paracetamol is 'if symptoms persist, consult a doctor.'

Minor and serious illness in African medicine

Although not formally so stated in TAM, traditional healers also practice their art in line with these two broad categories of illness. If an ailment fails to respond to well-known remedies, it is common sense that expert advice is sought.

In 1979, an important international workshop involving medical scientists and traditional healers was held at the famous Faculty of Pharmacy, University of Ife (now Obafemi Awolowo University) on the theme 'African Medicinal Plants', convened by the distinguished pharmacognosist Professor Abayomi Sofowora. The contributions of two highly respected Yoruba traditional healers on the issue of classes of illness in African medicine are instructive. Chief Labulo Apata[54] said:

> Medical herbalism (traditional African medicine) is divided into two branches: real treatment and psychological treatment. Real treatment is for those who require no incantations and other ceremonies. Psychological treatment . . . requires incantations and other ceremonies such as sacrifices before the medicine can act.

---

[54] L. Apata, The Practice of Herbalism in Nigeria. in: African Medicinal Plants, A. Sofowora, editor (Ile-Ife: University of Ife Press,1979) p. 16.

And, Chief J.O. Lambo[55] said that a traditional healer should know:

> How to trace five different causes of disease...
> (i) Physical ailments arising from poison, impurities or damage to any part of the body especially when it is localized; (ii) Psychological causes: when the will of man is not in harmony with the laws of nature, disease may follow... Unless these diseases are treated psychologically, no amount of drugs will effect cure; (iii) Astral influences: ....radiation from cosmic agents e.g. Sun, Moon and planets; (iv) Spiritual causes: diseases caused by all evil thoughts caused by passions, evil desires and machinations by enemies; (v) Esoteric causes: These are diseases springing from the soul e.g. insanity.

The difference between physical (minor ailments) and psychological (a serious life-threatening illness) in practice lies in whether the cause of discomfort is easily diagnosed or not. In a minor ailment, the cause of discomfort is, in the first instance, self-evident, for example, stomach upsets, cuts and bruises, bleeding, fractures, fever, aches and pains. The problem may be severe, but treatment is within the realm of common sense, that is, what has to be done to solve the problem, what has worked to produce cure in the past, is known. There is no anxiety as to whether the ailment was caused by 'psychological' supernatural agencies. In a 'psychological' illness (serious illness) the cause of what

---

[55] J.O. Lambo, The healing power of herbs, with special reference to obstetrics and gynaecology. in: Sofowora, op cit, p. 28.

might be imminent death is not known. In modern medical terminology, the cause may be an internal, serious disorder caused by cancer, cardiovascular failure, pneumonia, tuberculosis, kidney failure etc., where traditional healers cannot offer clear cut diagnoses. When they find that the usual treatments available for the cure of common ailments have failed, the people begin a search for clues that lie beyond common sense, by resorting to esoteric concepts and beliefs.

It is here that the difference between traditional and modern medicine is most manifest. The modern doctor conducts a scientific diagnosis consistent with the overarching germ theory of disease. Diagnosis here is the search for physical causes e.g., a malfunctioning heart/kidney/ liver/bladder, raised blood pressure etc. On the other hand, the African healer approaches a diviner for a supernatural explanation because in this culture the belief (theory) is that a supernatural agency may be responsible for the occurrence of severe illness. Both practitioners are acting rationally in search of the clues that require complex methods to reveal.

In African medicine, minor ailments are treated with plant preparations that are known from experience to possess the appropriate curative properties, e.g., freshly expressed leaf juices are used to arrest bleeding which may have been accidentally caused by scarification or circumcision. The beneficial effect of this treatment is due almost certainly to tannic acid or other haemostatic properties present in these plants. Tannic acid has protein-coagulating (astringent) properties and is widespread in the plant kingdom. Fever is a symptom of many disease conditions and is diagnosed by feel. A mother can tell that the baby on her back skin-to-skin is feverish from slight differences in their body temperatures. Diagnosis by feel is also what happens when, in the absence of a thermometer, one adult places his/her palm on another's forehead to diagnose fever. Anti-fever plants are consequently abundant in Nigerian cornucopia of medicine. According to the University of Ibadan eminent neurologist, late Professor Benjamin Osuntokun:

> The average Yoruba peasant . . . can recite recipes of herbs and concoctions that are supposed to relieve common symptoms. Most households have their favourite prescriptions for headache, fever and jaundice. [56]

I can corroborate this, as far as fever is concerned from a dramatic example that I obtained from Urhobo villages. In 2008, I asked first-year students of pharmacy at Delta State University, Abraka, to each bring a specimen of the plant most frequently used to treat fever in their respective villages. About half of the class of 27 students brought specimens of the shrub known in Urhobo as ubuko-iyeke, later identified for me at the University of Ibadan Herbarium as Phyllanthus amarus (family, Euphorbiaceae). The Urhobo use macerated ubuko-iyeke leaves (fresh or dried) in local gin to cure or prevent fever/'malaria'. Extracts of various species of Phyllanthus have been studied and found to contain

---

[56] B.O. Osuntokun, The traditional basis of neuropsychiatric practice among the Yoruba of Nigeria. Trop. Geogr. Med. 1975, (27): 412 - 30.

flavenoids and polyphenols[57] which are now known to possess a variety of anti-inflammatory and antioxidant properties.

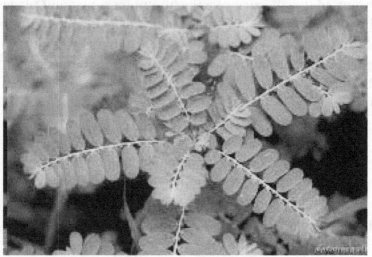

Phyllanthus amarus , local Urhobo name, ubuko-iyeke,

And, we know that plants used as anti-fever remedies have historically been sources of anti-inflammatory and anti-malaria drugs (salicin from willow bark, quinine from Cinchonna, artemisinin from quin hao (Artemesia annua), gedunin from dogon yaro (Azadirachta indica).[58]

In summary, treatment of minor ailments with herbal remedies in traditional medicine is in principle identical to the treatment of similar ailments with over the counter (OTC) medicines such as paracetamol in modern

---

[57] B. Oliver-Bever, Medicinal Plants in Tropical West Africa (Cambridge, Cambridge University Press, 1986), p. 169.

[58] See appendix 2. for a comprehensive review of anti-inflammatory mechanisms of action of plant remedies.

medicine. In both systems the medicine is used for its already recognized ability to cure the ailment.

Serious illness

For more complex ailments described by Chief Lambo as 'psychological' illnesses, where the cause of suffering is not obvious or cannot be ascertained from experience and the illness is protracted and life-threatening, a supernatural explanation is sought through divination.

An important point that needs to be stressed but which may not be obvious to some students of traditional medicine is this: In both traditional and modern medicine, the stage of the illness at which the practitioners consult 'higher realms' as it were, in search of a deeper understanding of causation is the stage when commonsense treatments (i.e., all treatments known from previous experience to be effective) have failed. It is at this stage that theoretical thinking takes over in both systems. In African medicine, the healer is engaged in a divinational search for answers from the supernatural, whereas scientific diagnosis in modern medicine is involved in a similar search among material invisible causes of illness---bacteria, viruses, parasites, dysfunctional organs or enzyme systems, etc., based on complex medical theories.

However, as discussed above, metaphysical explanations of illness causation in African medicine are not to be uncritically written off as nonsensical superstition. We have from authorities that 'from a historical point of view metaphysics can be seen to be the source from which the theories of empirical science spring.'[59]

What I am stressing here is that in life-threatening illnesses, divination in TAM and diagnosis in modern medicine are driven by the same impulses—to probe for clues to the cure of serious illness that lie beyond the range of common sense. What is it that we do not know from previous experience of treating common ailments that may kill the patient in this instance? Each (divination or scientific diagnosis) is rational in the culture and within the dogma/theory in which it operates. Historically, it was when metaphysical explanations of serious illness began to be replaced by rudimentary scientific explanations, that traditional European medicine began its development into what we now know as modern medicine. The proof of a scientific explanation demanded precise empirical data, which in turn demanded instrumentality and technology.

In Europe, the emergence of technology in the form of the microscope, gradually enabled the physical examinations (of live and post-mortem specimens) in search of the cause of illness or death, thereby, over time, replacing metaphysical explanations of illness. African societies remained isolated and out of range of the early science and technology developments taking place in Europe, hence metaphysical explanations of illness and death have persisted. A former University of Ibadan professor of veterinary pathology, T.T. Isoun has

---

[59] K. Popper, The Logic of Scientific Discovery 8th Impression (London, Hutchinson, 1975) p. 312.

pointed out,[60] that some traditional African peoples continue to perform

> . . . spiritual post-mortem examinations on
> their dead; they did not make the shift from a
> spiritual post-mortem to physical examination
> of the dead which could have advanced their
> concept of disease.

This is not to say that the religious constructs which attributed the occurrence of serious illness to supernatural causes in African medicine were irrational. It turns out that African ancients had very admirable intuitive insight into human nature which enabled them to evolve these explanations of illness that can now be seen as valid. The African insight into the causes of illness were not fundamentally different from those of the rest of humanity at similar levels of 'development'; that is, before science and technology brought about changes in the way we now understand illness.

Another point to stress here is that plants in traditional medicine are used in the treatment of serious illness for a variety of attributes, including their perceived 'occult power'[61] and not necessarily for their pharmacologically active chemical constituents. By 'occult power' Chief Lambo was probably expressing man's perception of plants as possessing extraordinary attributes. Plants reproduce in wondrous ways, possess healing and poisoning powers and they provide food and

---

[60] T. T. Isoun, Evolution of Science and Technology in Nigeria, The experience of the Rivers State University of Science and Technology. (Riverside Communications, Port Harcourt, 1978) p. 5.

[61] Lambo, p. 23.

shelter for man. Even science with its sophisticated technologies in chemistry, is unable to replicate the synthesis of some complex molecules found in plants. So it is not surprising that human beings have historically thought of plants as having 'supernatural powers'. Therefore one would be mistaken to expect a direct correspondence between traditional plant usage in the treatment of serious illness, and the pharmacologically active chemical constituents of the plant. In other words, if a traditional healer claims that a particular plant can 'cure' hypertension permanently, for example, the scientist should not rush to the conclusion that an extract of the plant must contain chemical entities with specific anti-hypertensive properties, because of the important question: "How does the traditional healer measure blood pressure without appropriate technology?"

Why there are no disease specialists in African medicine
Another aspect of African medicine that needs expatiation is the absence of disease or organ specialists. In modern medicine there are now numerous areas of medicine in which the doctor may specialize, such as in diseases of the cardiovascular system, renal, gastrointestinal, rheumatology, cancer, blood, skin, hair, teeth, etc. and further sub-subspecialties in these areas. This is because modern medicine defines illnesses in terms of specific physical causes and in terms of the organs of the body that are affected by the disease; and, there are the appropriate technologies that go with the specialties. Hence modern medicine is sometimes said to be guilty of being more interested in 'fighting the disease' than in caring for the ill person habouring the disease.

In African medicine, serious illness is defined holistically as a problem affecting the whole person; illness is understood, in Selye's terminology, as a manifestation of the body's struggle to adapt to stress, a nonspecific adaptation syndrome. In serious illness, a diffusion of emotional tension is an important therapeutic objective. Obviously therefore, traditional healers are not classified in terms of disease specialists in the way that modern medicine specialists are. Since emotional distress is considered a probable major contributor to the occurrence of serious illness, the methods that have the effect of restoring the sick person to emotional equilibrium are the important methods in African medicine and not treatments aimed at the elimination of specific physical causes of disease.

The nearest equivalent in traditional medicine is found in aspects of health care where the problem is clearly visible: for example some traditional healers are recognized as being more proficient at bone setting than others; birth attendance and associated skills are other areas where traditional healers and indeed many adults in traditional African societies possess competencies, which were acquired often by forced experience. A half brother of mine with many wives delivered his own children; he became so well known for the skill that he was often consulted by other members of his community when there was difficulty.

The specialists in African medicine are the herbalists and diviners who play important roles in diagnosis, prevention and treatment of illness.

a. Herbalists and herbal remedies

Traditional African healers are either predominantly practitioners of herbal medicine and/or diviners who are concerned with, and knowledgeable in, the art of uncovering spiritual underpinnings of serious illness. These two functions are known throughout Africa, but there is much variability in the extent to which the functions are separated among practitioners in different communities. The obo-epha's (diviner) role in the Urhobo tradition seems to be mainly divination, that is uncovering the spiritual hidden underpinnings of serious illness, whereas in some South African tribes the diviner, commonly a female (insangoma) may operate as such, as well as herbalist (inyanga).

Among the Yoruba it is said that,

". . . if you summon an Ifa priest (babalawo) to consult an oracle, after the appearance of odu . . . he may interpret and make mention of medicinal plants that were used for a similar (condition) in the past . . . this kind of plant is known as Ewe Ifa (a herb suggested by the Ifa oracle)".[62]

In other words, Ifa divination can reveal the cause of illness, as well as point to an appropriate plant remedy. In Yoruba medicine, another class of healer is the onisegun, who is a specialist in the use of herbs for various purposes.

Herbal remedies may be prepared and applied in many different ways. The oral route is commonly used:

---

[62] Apata, p. 16.

the plant part is macerated in hot or cold water, alcohol or palm wine, and a quantity of the liquid is taken as required; the fact that remedies are not taken in specified dosages as in modern medicine is often used to denigrate traditional medicine by biomedical scientists. But this is unjustified (see chapter 12, Dose of Medicine).

Topical application is also a common method in which, for example, the juice freshly squeezed from leaves may be applied directly to the affected part, e.g., to stop bleeding due to accidental injury or following circumcision. What are commonly called tribal marks, now rarely seen on Nigerian faces, were often scarifications for the application of medicine. Traditional African bone setters also use herbs in the 'plaster' encasement to aid mending/healing of the broken bone and in many different imaginative ways.

Traditional healers use plants to treat serious illness, but they may apply the preparations in non-pharmaceutical modes; for example, the preparation may be tied in a cloth/leather bundle and worn as amulet, anklet, waistband or necklace, or the bundle may be placed under the patient's pillow or sleeping mat or on the lintel of the door to the ill person's room. It is believed that remedies used in this way can be effective in curing or preventing internal ailments. I refer to this mode of plant remedies later in the chapter on the pharmacology of TAM and suggest that a rational explanation for any clinical benefits accruable to remedies so applied is the placebo mechanism, not magic (see chapter 13).

b. Diviners

Divination has been defined as a standardized process deriving from a learned discipline based on extensive body of knowledge. The diviner may utilize a fixed corpus such as the Yoruba Ifa Odu (verses) or a more diffuse body of esoteric knowledge.

In African medicine, divination is employed as diagnostic procedure for the detection of the supernatural underpinnings of a serious illness and for various other purposes that do not concern us here. Divination seems to have been an ancient practice in virtually every human community; it has been practised in India, Tibet, Indonesia and ancient Egypt. In Africa, divination is practised in Burkina Faso, Kenya, Madagascar, Uganda, Sierra Leone, Sudan, Togo, Congo, Zambia and in virtually every ethnic nationality in Nigeria. It is referred to as eva (Isoko); afa (Igbo); Ifa (Yoruba); epha (Urhobo). Most divination processes involve throwing down a set of objects and reading the pattern in which the objects lie in relation to one another. The diviner seems to be able to identify hidden stresses that underpin a serious illness or persons with evil intent (witches/wizards) and those transgressions that are capable of triggering ancestor spirit anger, from the position of the divining objects.

Among the Urhobo, when a problem—be it a serious life-threatening illness, consistent failure in business, infertility, etc.,—has defied every effort at resolution, the people consult a diviner (ke kpe epha, literally meaning 'they go to divination'). The following statement by

Michael Nabofa and Ben Elugbe[63] who have looked closely at Urhobo divination practices is of interest:

> Psychologists of religion, theologians and mystics have often tried to explain that wherever a mind is exposed in a spirit of absorbed submission to impressions of the universe, it becomes capable of experiencing intuition and feelings of the divine. In the thinking of the Urhobo it is such a mood that the diviner seeks to assume when he gazes meditatively at the instrument of divination during his practice. . . once he has attained a certain degree of attunement he . . . (can) tap useful information . . . from divine beings of the suprasensible world.

Urhobo diviners use many different instruments such as cowries, four-lobed kola nuts, coins of the same denomination, mirror, alligator pepper and different divination methods, but according to Nabofa and Elugbe, the most popular method and least likely to be 'rendered ineffective by negative rival forces is the agbragha apparatus' (made from the shells of the fruit of the agbragha tree).[64]

---

[63] M.Y. Nabofa and B.O. Elugbe, Epha: An Urhobo System of Divination and its Esoteric Language, in: Studies in Urhobo Culture, P.Ekeh, editor (Urhobo Historical Society, Monograph No. 2, 2005) p. 551.

[64] Ibid.

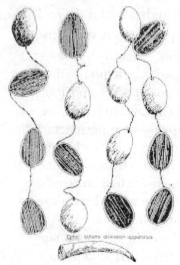

Agbragha divination shells.

Agbragha is made up of four divining chains (strings) each having four agbragha shells. Each shell is half of a round fruit which means that each shell has a convex side and a concave side. When the diviner throws down the sixteen shells, he has a computational riddle before him: How many of the four shells in each string lie with the concave side up and how many have the convex side up? Is it two of each, three of one and one of the other, etc? That is to say each of the four strings has infinite possibilities and therein lies the complexity of agbragha divination. The relative concave/convex positions of the shells in each string is a word in 'divination language'; all four strings must be thrown simultaneously, two in each hand, and the patterns in each string read; it is from the combination of all the words that the diviner makes his final pronouncement during repeated castings of the divination chains.

Matters are made more complex and mysterious by the fact that the 'word' represented by the concave/convex pattern of the shells is not an Urhobo word, but a word from a special epha lexicon which is unintelligible to the client and the ordinary Urhobo speaker; and which only those trained in agbragha divination can translate.

The interested reader may consult the paper by Michael Nabofa and Ben Elugbe under reference for fascinating details of this method of divination; the authors have analysed this 'language' and concluded that it is not a language as such but a collection of words, a lexicon that was most probably invented specifically for agbragha divination. The adept oboepha (diviner) must have in his memory the entire lexicon of hundreds of agbragha words and be able to recall the appropriate word that corresponds to the relative positions of

concave/convex shells in each string of the agbragha apparatus as described above. The only way an ordinary person can come to making sense of the workings of the agbragha divination apparatus is to think of it as a computer with a software programme that factors in all the variables and their probabilities.

Victor Turner, who studied ritual symbols among the Ndembu of Zambia, is of the view that the diviner tries to discover unconscious impulses behind antisocial behaviour:

> He feels after stresses and sore points in relationships, using the configuration of symbolic objects to help him concentrate on detecting the difficulties in configuration of real persons.[65]

He points out further that among the Ndembu the diviner plays a critically important role in consolidating social order and in reinforcing the moral values of society; and, because he operates in emotionally charged situations, the

---

[65] V. Turner, Drums of Affliction - A study of religious processes among the Ndembu of Zambia (London, IAP Hutchinson University for Africa, 1981) p. 45
.

moral norms of society are strikingly rehearsed repeatedly. My own observations among the Ughievwen corroborate this, and suggest that this may have been a universal function of divination in small-scale kinship societies.

Divination serves other important social purposes. The diviner's pronouncements often lead to libations and sacrifices being offered to the ancestors; in these, all members of the kinship group participate. The event often turns out to be a feast. Most of the food, drinks and cash offered in propitiation of angered ancestors (the so-called sacrifice) are shared and consumed by the participants. These activities have the effect of diffusing emotional tension all round, and at the same time restoring harmonious relationships between members of the group who were scandalized by the ill person's misdemeanour. Even if tensions are not totally diffused, the fact that the underlying stresses are exposed makes the relationship between members of the kinship group more tolerable.

c. Incantations

In African medicine, belief in the power of the word (ase, Yoruba; ota, Urhobo, for example) is highly entrenched; appropriately spoken words or incantation often accompany the collection of plant materials, the preparation of medicine and its administration, if the healing power of the medicine is to be realised.

Among Yoruba healers, each herbal medicine prescription may be accompanied by formally pronounced incantations, in which each component of the medicine and the illness to be treated is addressed. Such incantations are special verses (odus) from the corpus of Ifa, delivered evocatively and believed to be inspired by supernatural powers to activate the medication. Incantations are directed at the medicine and the illness, and indirectly at the emotional state of patient and caring kinship group; by thus pronouncing the appropriateness and potency of the treatment, incantation increases the efficacy of the therapy either by releasing the healing power of the plant (as traditional belief has it) or by a placebo mechanism. Incantation is medical poetry; in modern medicine, poetry (listening to it or writing it) has been shown to to have therapeutic benefit, as can visual art (appreciating it or creating it.)

Pierre Fatumbi Verger has recorded more than 400 tradi-tional healers' prescriptions among the Yoruba, each accom-panied by incantations; many of these being prescriptions to aid reproduction, including eight specifically for male virility. [66]

Medicine for virility

Root of Richiea caprodoides var. Longipedicellata (Cappara-caeae)

Ten whole fruits of Afromium melegueta (Zingiberacaceae)

Fruit of Musa sapientum var. Paradisiaca (Musacaceae)

Having peeled the banana, pound everything together. Grind. Draw the odu in the preparation and recite the following incantation. Drink with spirit or white corn meal.

---

[66] Pierre Fatumbi Verger, Ewe, the use of Plants in Yoruba Society (Sao Palo, Brazil, Odebrecht, 1995) see for example page 19.

The accompanying incantation is as follows:

Enisa oogun, help me apply medicine to my penis

Make it to be powerful

Ogede agbagba is always very powerful

Ataare is always very active.

Turner[67] recorded the following invocation of the Ndembu healers of Zambia when using parts of the mukula tree (Pterocarpus angolensis) for the treatment of infertility in women:

> The principal practitioner addresses the tree and says: 'Come o you mukula, isi kenu of women, who give birth in order to rear children' The practitioner then takes beer, pours libation and makes an invocation with it: 'Truly, give us our procreative power. Then he digs up the roots'.

Incantation is part of the evidence used in chapter eight on the pharmacology of TAM, that in traditional African thought, plants are perceived to have healing powers, a vital force (occult powers) which the incantation is believed to release. It seems perfectly reasonable that prescience societies attributed mystical powers to plants; plants are living things that reproduce in wondrous ways and sustain animal and human life. And as we know now they can make an extraordinary array of chemical entities, some curative some extremely poisonous! But an appropriately spoken incantation in an emotionally charged situation must have a calming and reassuring effect; and increase confidence in the treatment of serious illness; all these must contribute to the place.

---

[67] Turner, p. 59.

Chapter 7

Taboos and Witchcraft

T o fully appreciate that in traditional African medicine serious illness is viewed holistically as a catastrophe of community-wide proportions, it is important to explore the importance of beliefs other than those already described which are evoked in the treatment of an ill person. Adherence to other beliefs discussed in this section are apparently designed to prevent illness; they are beliefs whose functions in traditional society are to channel people away from behaviours that are most likely to provoke the occurrence of serious illness. These, along with incantations and divination methods already discussed above, constitute the paraphernalia of African medicine that biomedical scientists and western ethnographers most often describe in derogatory terms as superstition. This is almost certainly because there are no obvious equivalents of these beliefs in modern medicine; and, there appears to be no apparent rationale or reason for their deployment in the treatment of illness in modern medicine which is scientific evidence-based.

In this chapter I have picked out witchcraft and taboo beliefs that seem to have the attributes of preventive medicine for interrogation, to see if the deployment of these beliefs is consistent with the main objectives in African medicine, as elaborated upon in previous chapters.

I came to the conclusion that these beliefs, like the belief in ancestor spirit anger, underscore the critical linkage of antisocial/immoral behaviour to serious illness in traditional African thought; the overall conclusion from the analyses is that the operation of these beliefs had the effect of consolidating moral integrity in traditional African societies; taboo and witchcraft beliefs are basically moral laws that use the fear of sanction by the supernatural to enforce good moral conduct.

Taboos

A taboo is an act or thing which religion or custom forbids; in the African context, what enforces compliance with a taboo in the acculturated individual, is the belief that unpleasant consequences, induced by the supernatural, will follow its breach. Western thinkers have a tendency to brand taboos as irrational beliefs that serve no purpose. For example, Robin Horton considers that taboos are typically representative of the African mode of thinking:

> It is characteristic of taboo reaction that people are unable to justify it in terms of ulterior reasons: tabooed events are simply bad in themselves.[68]

---

[68]Patterns of Thought in Africa and the West (Cambridge, Cambridge University Press, 1993) p. 245.

This view of a taboo belief is typical of the unjustified way in which the western-trained mind sees taboos. As with African beliefs in general, a taboo belief is a religious dogma, its power lies in the expectations on the part of the acculturated individual, that a breach of the taboo will be punished by supernatural forces. Because of this religious configuration, believers in the taboo do not question this power; they do not question whether the symbolic figure of a fetish placed on farm produce has the power to punish a person who would steal the farm produce. The acculturated individual believes that it can, and that is where the power of the taboo lies. As with other traditional African beliefs that have to do with health, we can assume taboo beliefs are complex mnemonics embodying experiences gained over thousands of years and expressed as a shorthand statement, a metaphor. Again, the metaphor, being a religious construct, enables the belief to be used in socialization schemes for the moral upbringing of individuals in society.

My friend, the late Zack Ademuwagun, University of Ibadan Professor of Health Education, considered African taboos to be effective illness prevention laws, to preserve health; and, because there is a strong association between illness and antisocial behaviour in traditional African thought; taboos are also mechanisms for regulating moral conduct. To take some examples:

i. Sexual intercourse during a woman's menstrual period is taboo

Among many African peoples, it is forbidden, a taboo, for a man to have sexual intercourse with a woman during her menstrual period. Traditional practices designed to enforce compliance with this taboo, such as what amounts to monthly banning of the woman from her husband's bed, may appear like cruel punishment; in Urhobo for example, the euphemistic reference to a menstruating woman is orua uwovwin-i, literally meaning, she does not enter the house, i.e., the woman is in a state where she is not permitted to enter her husband's part of the household. This practice explains why in a typical Urhobo traditional household, a wife has her own room or quarters which she shares with her children; and in a polygamous household, each wife has her own separate living quarters. It is a testimony to the serious extent that some African societies took this taboo that men and women were prepared to put up with such harsh denial. It can be said that restrictions of this kind imposed by menstruation were a critical factor in the evolution of polygamy in many traditional African cultures.

Unpleasant consequences, it is believed, can flow from a breach of this taboo, for example, the woman may give birth to a child with a malformation such as albinism. The fear of such consequences may deter individuals from contravening the taboo, but the taboo's main significance may be hygiene. To prevent sexual intercourse at a time when the womb is thought to be vulnerable to damage. Also, prior to the advent of technology and modern developments in female hygiene, menstruation must have been a difficult time of the month when sexual intercourse might have been unpleasant and possibly harmful, to the male too. This taboo could have evolved to ensure that abstinence from sex during the menstrual period was religiously adhered to. The important point to stress is that we should not be too hasty in condemning traditional African beliefs and cultural practices before we have attempted to understand the circumstances in which those beliefs evolved.

ii. Female adultery is taboo in traditional African societies

It is forbidden in traditional African culture for a married woman to have extramarital sexual intercourse. "An act of adultery resulting in pregnancy must be confessed or else the woman would have difficulty during labour; if she delivers safely, she may lose the child or she herself may die during labour or after delivery", [69] (see also case 1, chapter 4, page 89). The fear of such potentially dreadful consequences may deter a married woman from committing adultery, but the real significance of this taboo is control of morality, and by extension, health. Among the Urhobo adultery by a married woman is emuerinvwin. This taboo, like others related to sexual behaviour that are heavily weighted against the female, was obviously invented by the male in traditional human societies. However, what may appear on the face of it to be crass 'male chauvinism' was most probably in reality the genetic urge of the male to protect his woman, the bearer of his children and the genetic integrity of his lineage from violation by another male predator.

---

[69] Z. Ademuwagun, 1984, personal communication.

iii. Magun

The Yoruba have one taboo that has the effect of deterring men from chasing after married women. It is called magun literally meaning 'do not climb'.

> Magun is medicine applied to a woman suspected to be promiscuous by her husband, so that any man other than the husband who climbs her may experience a number of hardships, including inability to withdraw from the woman or the man may die during intercourse.[70]

We must note here that adultery was taboo for a married woman in traditional African culture where polygamy was more the rule than the exception; in most of these societies male adultery i.e., intercourse with a woman who is not his wife would be frowned upon by some, but it was not a serious sin, unless the relationship was incestuous, in which case it is an abomination. But the Yoruba have invented magun to deter male adultery specifically involving a married woman.

An important issue arises as to whether magun medicine has inherent powers to kill as described or whether magun's ability to deter is the belief itself. For those brought up to believe in magun this distinction is academic. In the accult-urated individual, belief per se is a sufficient deterrence. Since the man would not know which married woman is protected by magun, the safe thing would be to avoid intercourse with any married woman. Therein lies the power of magun to deter men from chasing after married women.

---

[70] Ibid.

An interesting conversation between Chief Obafemi Awolowo (Awo)[71] and the University of Ife (now Obafemi Awolowo University) philosopher, Professor Moses Akin Makinde (Mak) on magun is worth recalling here.[72]

The question was: Is magun real? If a man commits adultery with a married woman and dies on top of her during sexual intercourse, is magun the only explanation for his death? Here is a short fragment of the exchange:

> Awo – "The truth about magun is this. When a man has heart trouble, he can die while making love to any woman. I have known two cases for certain of those who were reported to have died of magun, when in actual fact they died of heart attack right on top of women, having sex . . . ."
>
> Mak – "So he died just like that, of sex?"
>
> Awo –"Of course, that was what he loved, and that was what killed him. The doctor asked him to rest, and he died working on his concubine . . . ."

Chief Awolowo was clearly not convinced that magun has an intrinsic power to kill. His argument is similar to that of the empirical thinker who wants an objective proof that magun can kill. In countering the chief, the professor evoked a philosophical concept "the principle of rationality which is used in Games and Decisions Theory. Under this principle you are making a choice

---

[71] Chief Obafemi Awolowo (1909-1987) was the legendary first premier of the Western Region, Nigeria.

[72] M.A. Makinde, Awo. The Last Conversation (Ibadan, Evans Brothers, 2010) p. 167-174.

(between alternatives) under uncertainty of outcomes".
The professor argues as follows:

> Mak - "Now, if you are rational and you
> maximize your expected utility, you will
> choose not to have sex with a woman laid with
> magun precisely because of the outcome of a
> decision you have taken under uncertainty
> about whether or not magun kills. By
> maximizing my expected utility therefore, my
> rational decision will then be, don't do it . . .
> Therefore, if I am asked to choose between a
> belief in magun or no magun when nobody has
> proved or disproved scientifically that magun
> is efficacious, I will choose to believe that it
> may be a killer and so run away from it . . . .
> That is precisely the message of maximization
> of expected utility and the wager argument
> concerning the magun hypothesis."

The chief was not entirely convinced by the professor's
philosophical argumentation but concedes a point:

> Awo - "That is interesting, but in the case of
> magun because we don't experiment over it, I
> don't trust what people say about it . . . You
> have made your point on the basis of what will
> happen to you if you sleep with a woman laid
> with magun . . . ."

I have reproduced this exchange here because it
essentially represents the positions of the empirical
scientist who demands experimental proof prior to
acceptance of a hypothesis, and that of the philosopher;
Professor Makinde's position agrees with the general
trend I have taken in this book, that in traditional
African culture, belief in itself has potency; even those

who may be sceptical about the intrinsic power of magun to kill, may be deterred from chasing married women, just in case. The belief is religious. The reality or existence of the enforcer, magun, is accepted in faith.

Witchcraft belief

Witchcraft belief is widespread in Africa. Witches/wizards are persons with extraordinary powers to do evil—to cause illness and death and other misfortunes. Sir Edward Evans-Pritchard's study of witchcraft belief among the Azande of the Sudan is probably the most authoritative of its kind on the subject. He published the classic Witchcraft, Oracles and Magic among the Azande in 1937. He wrote that

> . . . an act of witchcraft is a psychic act, involving no ritual performance, spell utterance or medicines.

In this respect witchcraft differs from sorcery which relies on the use of powerful medicines or spells to cause harm[73] Witchcraft can take place across immense distances. Time, gravity and space are no barriers to a determined witch/wizard. The Urhobo word for witch/wizard, oriedan literarily meaning "she/he knows how to fly" summarizes the perception that witches have extraordinary powers. A tragic sudden death, failure in life in general, failure at particular endeavours, protracted illness, etc. are the kinds of misfortunes usually attributed to the machinations of witchcraft,

---

[73] See P.J. Imperatto, African Folklore Medicine Practices and Beliefs of the Bambara and other Peoples (New York Press, Baltimore 1977), for descriptions of poisonous potions used by Bambara sorcerers of Mali).

although when it comes to serious protracted illnesses
and death therefrom, diviners may also search for sins
capable of triggering ancestor spirit anger. Evans-
Pritchard [74]wrote that witchcraft beliefs also embrace a
system of values designed to regulate human behaviour:

> The concept of witchcraft provides a natural
> philosophy by which the relations between
> men and unfortunate events are explained and
> a means of reacting to events . . . behaviour
> which conflict with Zande ideas of what is right
> and proper, though not in itself witchcraft,
> nevertheless is the drive behind it, and persons
> who offend against the rules of conduct are
> most frequently exposed as witches.

It is from the perspective that witchcraft belief has an
inherent behaviour control function that the belief has
relevance in African medicine; in which serious illness is
critically linked to antisocial/immoral conduct. It seems
that in general, traditional African religious beliefs have
both health and moral connotations, which raises the
likelihood discussed earlier on (in chapter 3, pages 65-
66) that the impulse that drove the evolution of beliefs
such as the witchcraft belief, was the imperative for strict
moral behavior and conformity with social norms by
members of the kinship group. Evans-Pritchard also
makes the point that:

> The notion of witchcraft is not only a function
> of misfortune and of personal relations but it
> also comprises moral judgment ... Hatred,

---

[74]Witchcraft, Oracles, and Magic among the Azande (Oxford, Clarendon Press,
1937) p. 109.

> jealousy, envy, backbiting, slander etc, go forth
> ahead and witchcraft accusations follow.[75]

It seems that witchcraft belief is another traditional African doctrine whose "purpose" was to ensure adherence to accepted societal norms; the belief could deter individuals from engaging in behaviour most likely to provoke accusations of witchcraft which had serious consequences in traditional African societies.

Even though the witchcraft belief might have evolved with the puritanical purpose of controlling morality, the belief has been subjected to, and most probably corrupted by socio-political realities in African societies over the years. Since the consequences of being accused of witchcraft are dire, including shame for the family of the accused or death by ordeal poisoning or out right murder of the accused, witchcraft belief became a weapon in the hands of traditional authority: In Ibibio/Efik societies where the Calabar bean (etu esere bean) was used as ordeal poison (see chapter 9 below), the poison was administered by high ranking medicine men: the mbia-indiong and mbia-ibok; persons accused of witchcraft were thus more likely, than not, to be the peasantry. Similarly, among the Azande, witchcraft accusation and detection occurred more frequently among the commoners than among the princes who ruled the clans.[76] I found no evidence of obvious class distinction in witchcraft accusation among the

---

[75] Ibid.

[76] E. Gilles, E. E. Evans-Pritchard. Witchcraft, Oracles, and Magic among the Azande (Oxford, Clarendon Press, 1976).

Ughievwen community where traditional society was a classless peasantry of village republics. What is apparent from general observation is that the poor and elderly are more likely to be victims of witchcraft accusations than the rich and famous who tend more and more, to keep themselves and their children away from the villages where the poor and elderly reside.

Even though the positive morality control function of witchcraft belief is not openly expressed, there is evidence in Ughievwen society that the poor and elderly who recognize that they are the most likely victims of witchcraft accusations usually try to conduct themselves in such a way (like going to church) as to avoid witchcraft accusations. In every part of Nigeria, though, where the belief is still strong, witchcraft is seen as pure evil and those suspected to be witches are subjected to harsh inhumane punishments or even killed by their relatives, despite the fact that no objective evidence has ever been proffered for the existence of witchcraft as a reality. Such is the power of belief.

The curse

Another belief that is recognized as having a bearing on serious illness is the curse. To curse someone is to wish evil to happen to that person; that wish being uttered verbally or symbolically. In traditional African societies, it is believed that serious illness or death can arise from a curse. This belief is widespread in Africa—from among the Urhobo and Yoruba in Nigeria to the Creole and Mende of Sierra Leone. A curse pronounced by an elder is believed to be potent, especially if the circumstances are such that the elder was considered justified in evoking the curse in the first place, i. e., the person cursed was adjudged by the kinship group to deserve the curse, being guilty of failure to render a traditional obligation to the elder, e.g., a son fails to support his aged poor parents; even though every one can see that the son is wealthy enough to help them, he deliberately allows them to suffer.

A mother's curse is greatly feared by her children who must therefore avoid the possibility of such provocation. A curse is usually delivered in the form of well chosen words addressed directly to the victim or as a symbolic ritual, in the absence of the victim; it may also be in the form of medicine such as magun applied by a jealous husband on a promiscuous wife, or an object placed on a farm to indicate that any one who steals the farm produce will suffer dire consequences. It may also be in the form of an object placed across the road or passage, such that if the intended victim crosses the object, serious illness or death may happen.

Professor Sawyerr considers that the appellation of magic sometimes applied to the effect of a curse is inappropriate; the term magic suggests an illusion, whereas the ill effects of a curse are real. Sawyerr [77] puts the point as follows:

> The effect of a curse on man within the African
> context is not due to magic but to a conflict

---

[77] H. Sawyerr, An inquiry into some aspects of psychic influence in African understanding of life. in: Themes in African Social and Political Thought, O Otite, editor (Enugu, Fourth Dimension Publishers,1978) p.73.

which is psychological in nature, created by
fear of sin committed against the sensus
communis ... which gnaws into the psychic life
of the offender thereby causing him to be ill.

If a mother's curse uttered in agony produces the
expected effect, e.g., the son becomes seriously ill it
would be, in my interpretation, because the son had
harboured the knowledge of his guilt for failure to
perform his traditional obligation to his mother,
according to his upbringing. It is the accumulated
experience of this kind that led to the evolution of the
belief in the power of the curse; thus the belief could
regulate social/moral conduct in suitably acculturated
members in traditional African society.

In concluding this section, we can say that for the
acculturated individual, the power of the curse to control
behaviour comes from the unquestioning belief in its
potency, and this seems to apply to other traditional
religious beliefs, such as witchcraft, taboo, ancestor spirit
anger, etc; these beliefs seem to have evolved with the
purpose of ensuring that members of the kinship group
behave in a moral and socially acceptable way.

In general we may suggest as follows from what we
have discovered so far: a serious life-threatening illness
was a symptom of antisocial/immoral conduct in African
thought; the sin must be confessed, and appropriate
sacrifices made before the individual can expect to regain
good health. Through serious illness in a member of the
kinship group, one might suggest, the ancestors drew
attention of the kinship group to an abomination by one
of their member which, if not appropriately treated,

could threaten harmony and cohesion of the group. Thus a serious illness in one member was a threat to all members; hence, once the illness was serious enough to compel divination consultation, it would have assumed a kinship group-wide concern. It seemed that proper moral conduct was of utmost importance: Immorality/antisocial behaviour was to be avoided at all costs. I hold the view that the beliefs described in this chapter evolved to ensure that members of small-scale African kinship groups adhered to a strict moral code of behaviour which was considered crucial for the harmonious survival of such societies.

Chapter 8

Herbs and Drugs as Therapeutic Tools: Pharmacology viewed from the perspective of traditional medicine

T he aspect of traditional African medicine that comes close to making sense to modern medical science is the use of herbal remedies. This is because plants have been known for centuries to be a source of medicines; plants yield many of the drugs that are used in modern medicine today. African medicinal plants are thus seen in modern medicine circles as potential sources of commercially profitable drugs. My contention is that the use of plant remedies in African medicine cannot be fully understood nor can the potential of African medicinal plants as source material for drugs be fully realized, without understanding the methods and esoteric beliefs that underlie their use in TAM.

So far in this book, I have treated these beliefs as the theoretical framework for TAM practices, and concluded that over all, TAM practices are consistent with the core belief that serious illness has its origins in emotional turmoil, and that the restoration of a seriously ill person to a state of emotional equilibrium is an important objective of therapy. Following from that, plant remedies ought to be evaluated, not merely as the equivalent of drugs used in modern medicine, but as components of the ritual processes employed in the holistic management of serious illness. The difference between drugs and herbal medicines is made clear by explaining that a drug is a pure chemical substance of natural or synthetic origin, having well-defined specific actions, and can be used to treat disease. The use of drugs in modern medicine is so important that a separate branch of medical science, pharmacology, is devoted to their study; drug discovery and development are based on theories and methods elaborated in pharmacology. It will therefore help our understanding of the differences between drugs as used in modern medicine and herbal remedies as they are used in TAM to briefly define some essential properties of drugs and to sketch some basic principles of pharmacology.

Pharmacology

Pharmacology is the discipline concerned with the complex mechanisms by which drugs bring about beneficial and sometimes harmful effects in man (and animals), and the processes by which drugs are removed from the body. These are highly complex issues involving vast numbers of scientists and disciplines in universities, research institutes and the pharmaceutical industry worldwide. Drugs are pure chemical substances and form a critically important part of therapy either to cure/control disease or as adjunct to other forms of medical intervention, such as surgery, anesthesia, etc. Many drugs interact very specifically and characteristically with biological systems and are therefore tools for delineating biochemical and physiological phenomena. The importance of drugs in medicine is underscored by the fact that pharmacology is a mandatory subject in the curricula for the training of doctors, pharmacists, nurses, etc.

Pharmacology as a theory of selective poisoning for therapeutic purposes

The central most important idea in pharmacology is that a drug, to be any good, must bind with high affinity, selectively, to the cause of disease and be able to prevent the cause from producing the symptoms of the disease, whether the cause is an enzyme, receptor, parasite, bacterium, fungus, virus, cancer, etc. In other words, the drug is designed to selectively discern the cause of disease, a theory usually referred to as selective toxicity (elaborately enunciated in Professor Adrien Albert's classic book, Selective Toxicity. The physico-chemical basis of therapy.[78]

The idea of selective toxicity can be traced to the discovery by Ehrlich (often referred to as the father of the science of chemotherapy) at the turn of the 19th century, that when dyestuffs are injected into living animals, some classes of dyes stain certain organs or

---

[78] (London ,Chapman and Hall, 1951).

tissues more specifically than other tissues, while other dyes are more general in their binding; for example, certain groups of dyes including methylene blue stain nervous tissues rather selectively. Ehrlich later discovered that in the same way, synthetic or naturally occurring chemical substances could selectively bind to, and kill, or stop the growth of disease-causing agents (parasites, bacteria, etc.) in the body. The chemical entity then acted like a magic bullet, selectively hitting the disease-causing parasite and interfering with its vital biochemical functions and killing it, without harm to the cells of the person infected by the pathogen.

The theory has been hugely successful in guiding the production of drugs for the treatment of many human and animal diseases: Scientists have found numerous existential biochemical systems in disease-causing microorganisms which can be blocked to kill the organism or prevent its growth without harming host cells, e.g., chloroquine can selectively kill the malaria parasite, Plasmodium falciparum, without harming the normal cells in the body of the patient. The theory has been extended to drugs for the treatment of non-infectious diseases also, e.g., hypertension, Parkinson's disease, Alzheimer's disease, psychoses, cancer, diabetes etc,—where the targets are for example, essential malfunc-tioning enzymes, abnormally growing cells, malfunctioning neurotransmitters and receptor systems. Tremendous advances in biochemistry, physiology, molecular biology and genetics in the last few decades have led to the discovery of an incredible range of receptor macromolecules and their selectively binding drugs (agonists and antagonists), thereby enabling pharmacologists to apply the theory of selective toxicity to the development of a wide range of drugs for disease control. Drug receptors, described by Professor H.P. Rang, President of the British Pharmacological Society, as pharmacology's big idea are the fundamental vehicles by which selective toxicity is achieved.

The traditional healer/herbalist, if forced to think about it, would describe pharmacology as a theory of selective poisoning for therapeutic purposes. That description would be inadequate for a professional pharmacologist, but it is accurate and appropriate for the present discussion; it enables us to make the distinction between drugs in modern medicine and plant remedies in African medicine. The major preoccupation in pharmacology today is the discovery of chemical substances that can selectively kill or substantially modify the causative agent, without harm to the patient. A good drug is one with a high selective toxicity for the cause of disease.

No matter how refined drug discovery processes have become in recent years, it is in the nature of biological systems that absolute selectivity cannot be guaranteed; hence all drugs have side effects (usually due to the actions of the drug on structures other than the intended target); most side effects are undesirable, some are fatal. In fact, the term 'pharmacology' is derived from the

Greek word pharmakon which means 'poison' in classic
Greek, and 'drug or medicine', in modern Greek.[79]

The idea that poisons can be used as medicines was
recognized more than 2000 years ago when the metal
arsenic was first used as therapy in traditional European
medicine. The 16th century Swiss physician, Paracelsus
Theophrastus von Hohenheim (also famous for
inventing the doctrine of signatures is quoted as saying
that 'all (chemical) substances are poisons' —the right
dose differentiates a poison from a remedy.[80]

Different treatment objectives: Modern medicine and
traditional African medicine

In traditional medicine, restoration of the patient to
emotional equilibrium, rather than the poisoning of a
specific causative agent is the major therapeutic objective
in the treatment of serious illness where sustained
emotional distress is perceived to be an important
causative factor. So, even though herbal remedies are
used in the treatment of serious illness in TAM (as are
drugs in modern medicine) the targets are different;
while drugs target an identified cause of disease for
elimination or modification, plant remedies as used in
TAM are best understood as therapeutic adjuncts in the
holistic management of serious illness where the overall
aim is to diffuse emotional tension.

---

[79] P. Routledge, Murder, mystery, medicine and their practitioners, Pharmacology
Matters /Newsletter, August 2011: 23-24.

[80] Ibid.

Even if one could convince the traditional healer that the cause of illness was, say, cancer, diabetes or tuberculosis, he would insist that there was an underlying more remote cause before the cancer, for example, emotional upheaval (emuerinvwin) which made the particular individual suscept-ible to the illness. In traditional African thought the remote cause is a legitimate therapeutic target.[81]

African pharmacopoeia of plant remedies

If we say that in general, diffusion of emotional tension, rather than the specific poisoning of a cause of disease, is the main objective in the management of serious illness in TAM, and that the placebo effect is a reasonable explanation for the clinical benefit of herbal remedies used in these conditions (see the chapter 13 on the placebo phenomenon below), then certain questions arise: For example, what kinds of plants do we expect the pharmacopoeia[82] of African remedies to consist of? In other words, should we really expect the plant remedies used to treat serious illness in TAM to work like drugs in modern medicine? We know that in the latter, the objective is to use the drug to specifically render the

---

[81] D.T. Okpako, Traditional African Medicine: Theory and pharmacology explored. Trends in Pharmacological Sciences 1999, 20: 482B 484; Idem, Good Drugs Don't Grow on Trees or Do They? (Ibadan, Ibadan University Press, 1988) 30pp; Idem, Malaria and Indigenous Knowledge in Africa, (Ibadan, Ibadan University Press, 2011).

[82] By 'pharmacopoeia' I mean the informal body of plants from which traditional healers and traditional African communities select their remedies for the treatment of minor ailments or serious life-threatening illnesses. This pharmacopoeia circulates in traditional societies by word of mouth and is passed on from generation to generation.

cause of disease dysfunctional or to kill it; the ideal drug is one that can do this without harm to the patient. In the treatment of serious illness in TAM, the target is not a physical cause to be eliminated with a poison (drug), but restoration of the patient to emotional equilibrium and harmony with his environment, so that the patient's body can heal itself. Fortuitously, as I demonstrate below, what constitutes the pharmacopoeia of the plants used in TAM as remedies excluded poisonous plants.

It is common knowledge that many of the important drugs used in modern medicine today were derived from poisonous plants. Such plants are usually known to indigenous African communities, but the people do not, as a rule, use them for healing purposes. So, that is partly the answer to the questions posed at the head of the last paragraph: the corpus of remedies for the treatment of serious illness in TAM is a pharmacopoeia which, as a rule, does not include plants that are known to be overtly poisonous; the plants normally used as therapy in TAM should not, in all probability, be expected to yield poisonous molecules with the potential for development into drugs with high selective toxicity.

Here incidentally is therefore an important lesson for those searching for drugs in African medicinal plants: The chances of discovering chemical entities with drug-like properties for the treatment of serious diseases like cancer, cardiovascular disease, etc., are better, if the search focuses on poisonous plants that are not used by indigenous healers as therapy, than if the search focuses on herbal remedies used regularly for healing purposes.

There is evidence for this view from research carried out by the American National Cancer Institute many years ago which showed that anti-cancer activity (the ability of the plant extract to selectively kill cancer cells) was significantly higher in extracts from poisonous plants than in extracts from plants actually used by indigenous people for the treatment of cancer;[83] see also a recent review of Chinese medicine.[84]

Two separate factors may account for the emergence of a pharmacopoeia of plant remedies that excluded overtly poisonous plants: The first factor is absence of precision technology in African cultures. As I have alluded to already, the availability of precision technology was decisive in enabling poisons to be used as drugs in modern medicine; with precision technology, quantities (weights and volumes) could be determined accurately in absolute units, and so could time. This meant that the quantity of the poison required for a therapeutic effect with minimum toxic side effects could be determined. Precision technology also permitted a drug's other quantitative formulation parameters, that is, the drug's average therapeutic dose in man, its pharmacokinetic profile and the time interval between doses for optimum therapeutic effect, to be determined.

Although the concepts of weight, volume and time exist in traditional African cultures, African societies

[83] B. Holmstedt and J.C. Bruhn, Is there a place for ethnopharmacology in our time? Trends in Pharmacological Sciences 1982 (3): 181-183.

[84] S. Man, W.Gao, C. Wei, and C. Liu, Anticancer drugs from traditional toxic Chinese medicines, Phyotherapy Research 2012 (26): 1449 B 1465.

were isolated from the precision technology revolution taking place in Europe, which enabled these concepts to translate into measurements in absolute units in those societies; in African cultures the concepts are applied in relative terms, such that to know which of two yams is heavier, you 'weigh' each by feel in each hand, if the difference is not clear by eye. To know which of two boys is taller, you stand them back to back. Even today in Nigerian markets commodities such as rice, egusi, pepper, elubo or garri, are sold in units of baskets or calabashes or kongos, which are imprecise measures of volume, for items that should be sold by weight.[85] Time is a complex idea in traditional African thought that we cannot go into here except to say that the day in traditional Africa consisted of day break, afternoon and night time; the modern 24 hour clock divided into hours, minutes, seconds and fractions of a second is a product of the recent precision technology which did not exist in the cultures in which TAM evolved. To deal with this conundrum in TAM, traditional societies, fortuitously perhaps, evolved a pharmacopoeia of plant remedies that excluded overtly poisonous plants.

The other reason why the exclusion of poisonous plants from the African pharmacopoeia of plant remedies is understandable is that the therapeutic target in the use of these remedies to treat serious-life threatening illness does not require the use of poisonous

---

[85] Okpako, Good Drugs Don't Grow on Trees or Do They? op cit.

plants, which as we shall see, are the usual plant sources of drugs now commonly in use in modern medicine.

To repeat what has already been said for emphasis, the overarching principle in TAM is that serious illness has its origins in the mind of the sufferer. Hence a major therapeutic objective is the diffusion of emotional tension, and not the incapacitation or the poisoning of a specific cause of disease. Indigenous African communities knew poisonous plants which they used as arrow poison,[86] fish poisons, ordeal poisons (for witchcraft detection), or poisons to dispose of an enemy. As a general rule, traditional healers deliberately avoid the use of poisonous plants as remedies in the treatment of illness. I am informed that in Yoruba culture, traditional healers are specifically forbidden, on ethical grounds, from using what they know to be poisonous in their healing practices (Femi Fatoba, personal communication, 1984).

It was fortuitous that the pharmacopoeia of plant remedies that evolved in TAM excluded poisonous plants; traditional medicine could not have succeeded in Africa otherwise.

---

[86] The term curare which describes various South American arrow poisons is used conventionally as reference to compounds with muscle relaxing properties. Arrow poisons are known worldwide, but their use by the Indians of the Amazon and Orinoco River basins attracted the attention of the explorer, Sir Walter Raleigh, who brought curare to Europe in the 16th century. Native South Americans made their curare from various species of Strychnos, e.g., Strychnos toxifera which contains toxiferine, the most potent of all curare alkaloids. Chlorodendron tomentosum is the plant source of the drug tubocurarine, widely used in modern medicine as muscle relaxant.

We can say that just as precision technology was necessary for the successful use of poisons in modern drug therapy, so was the exclusion of poisonous plants from the repertoire of plant remedies, necessary for the successful use of plant remedies in TAM.

Evolution of a poison-free pharmacopoeia of plant remedies

The two factors discussed above, namely, the absence of precision technology and the selective toxicity principle, are a good hindsight explanation for the exclusion of poisonous plants from the TAM repertoire of medicinal plants. But these factors could not have counted as prima facie considerations in the evolution of a poison-free pharma-copoeia; precision technology and the selective toxicity theory were unknown to African ancients, and could obviously not have been factors on which their selection of medicinal plants was based.

We can only speculate on what drove the evolution of a poison-free pharmacopoeia of plant remedies in TAM: The ancients, most probably, selected medicinal plants the same way as they selected food plants—on the basis of physical characteristics (appearance, smell, taste, flavour, color etc,) certainly, not on the consideration of the pharmacology of their chemical constituents. They could have discovered which plants were poisonous from experience of being poisoned by the plant; for example, when they experimented with the use of the plant as food or medicine. If the plant caused overt undesirable effects, they would have abandoned its use either as food or medicine and over time such poisonous plants would be known and avoided. This probably explains why it is the case that many of the plants used as remedies in TAM are also items of food, e.g., spices, food vegetables, flavoring agents, food preservatives and condiments.

Many plants contain extremely bitter tasting and poisonous substances, thought to have evolved to protect them against predation and disease pests. It is reasonable to presume that during the thousands of years during which man relied on plants for food and medicines, plants with a nasty taste or odor or that proved to be overtly poisonous, when consumed by accident or trial, were identified and avoided in future encounters (e.g., poisonous mushrooms and poisonous yams). Where the plant part looked as if it would be a valuable item of food (e.g., a hefty tuber, Dioscorea rotundata, or cassava), indigenous people found ways to remove the poison or nasty taste. For example, cassava (Manihot esculenta); burrawangs (Alocasia macrorhizos and Macrozamia spp), are staple foods of sub-Saharan Africans and Australian Aborigines respectively; these have to be specially processed to remove the poison before their use as food. In the case of cassava the extremely bitter taste of the tuber is due to the cyanogenic glycoside, a precursor of the highly poisonous hydrogen cyanide.

Cassava undergoes elaborate processing to render it safe for human consumption. In 1968, University of

Ibadan neurologist Benjamin Osuntokun[87] showed that the habitual c consumption of inadequately processed cassava, combined with inadequate protein intake, caused ataxic peripheral neuropathy, a chronic neurological disease common in some parts of Nigeria and recognized by the Ijebu (a subgroup of the Yoruba) as rase rase. The Ijebu had correctly associated the condition with excessive consumption of poorly processed garri (Dr. Olu Olusanya, personal communication 2010).

Let me conclude this section by reiterating that in traditional African medicine, overtly poisonous plants tended to be excluded from their repertoire of remedies. This made sense in the context of what I have referred to as the core principle in African medicine: in the treatment of serious illness, what was needed was a poison-free repertoire of plant remedies that could be used in holistic combination with ritual performance to diffuse emotional tension; for this purpose the remedy could be used without adherence to strict rules of dosage. Whereas in modern medicine, poisonous plants have been an important sources of drugs, consistent with the germ theory of disease in which the aim of therapy is to selectively poison the cause of disease. The availability of precision technology was crucial for success in the use of poisonous substances as drugs; in this, strict adherence to the rules of dosage is mandatory.

---

[87] B.O. Osuntokun, An ataxic neuropathy in Nigerians. A clinical, biomedical, and electrophysiological study. Brain, (91) 1968: 215.

What I have referred to here tentatively as non poisonous plants from the TAM pharmacopoeia, could be used safely and imaginatively and applied in unorthodox ways. See Chapter 12 on Dose of Medicine, where I argue that the usual criticism of TAM on the grounds that the practice is dangerous and invalid because its medicines are not prescribed in doses as drugs are in modern medicine, is inappropriate.

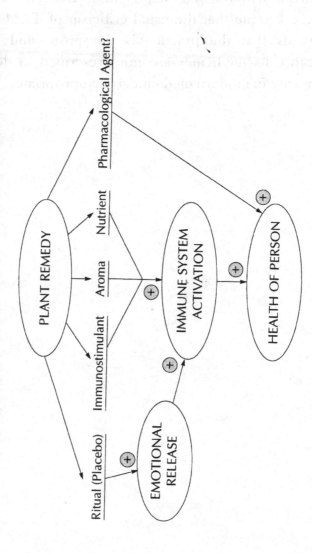

HOW PLANT REMEDIES WORK IN TRADITIONAL AFRICAN MEDICINE

Chapter 9

The Calabar Bean: A traditional African poison that yielded a famous drug

I n this chapter, I wish to tell the story of the famous etu esere bean of Calabar as a classic example of a plant material that was known to indigenous people to be highly poisonous, and avoided by them as therapy, but which yielded an important drug in modern medicine. The story of physostigmine is known to every undergraduate in the medical and pharmaceutical sciences. I have retold aspects of it here because of its significance in the context of traditional African medicine. How did the Ibibio/Efik indigenous people discover the poison and, remarkably, how did they link its unique pharmacological properties to witchcraft detection? And, we know that physostigmine turned out to be one of the most important medical discoveries of the 19th century.

Textbooks of pharmacology and medicine usually credit the discovery of physostigmine to the University of Edinburgh doctor, T.R. Fraser, who first extracted the alkaloid from the Calabar bean, but not many people know that the pharmacological properties of esere bean, used for centuries in southeastern Nigeria for witchcraft detection, were first discovered by the Ibibio and Efik people of present day Akwa Ibom and Cross River States. As is usual in Africa, the point of contact with Europeans when documentation began tends to be seen as the beginning of our history. In this case, the years of observation, trials and experience that resulted in esere bean becoming approved by the people as a reliable substance for witchcraft detection, were ignored and forgotten.

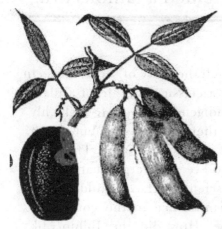

Physostigmine (eserine)

The important drug, physostigmine or eserine, comes from the seeds of the climbing plant Physostigma venenosum (Calabar bean), also known in Ibibio/Efik as etu esere. The ancient medicine men from this part of Nigeria (now Akwa Ibom and Cross River States) discovered that the esere bean had the power to 'reveal and destroy witchcraft'.

The British colonial officers who witnessed the dramatic -manifestations of etu esere in public during witchcraft ordeal trials were duly impressed. They took specimens of the bean to the United Kingdom and in 1840 Dr. T.R. Fraser of the University of Edinburgh began a detailed scientific investigation and published a gold medal-winning MD thesis on The pharmacological properties and therapeutic uses of the ordeal bean of Calabar.[88]

Concerning the Ibibio/Efik society of that time, Fraser wrote:

---

[88] T.R. Fraser, On the characters, actions and therapeutical uses of the bean of Calabar (Physostigma venenosum, Balfour). Edinburgh Medical Journal (1863) (9): 36-56.

The government is oligarchical. Several chiefs
rule the towns, each of which separately forms
an independent government, joining with
others in times of danger for the common
cause, and possessing with them a common
council. This is presided over by one of their
number and who on this account receives the
title King. . . . Next in power are the medicine
men—mbia idiong and mbia ibok. In their
conditions of ignorance, superstition reigns
supreme. Everything inexpli-cable—sorrow,
disease and death—are ascribed to the
mysterious agency of witchcraft. And it is for
the discovery of the operations of this evil
genius that the discriminating power of the
ordeal bean is required.[89]

The charge of witchcraft was made before a chief who then
summoned a meeting of the council of chiefs to hear the
charge and the defence of the accused. The individual
usually opted for the ordeal test. This consisted of infusion
made from ground esere bean and administered in public
view, watched by a crowd of onlookers. The infusion was
administered in increasing amounts until the accused
vomited (proof of innocence) or collapsed and died (proof
of guilt). In Fraser's account of his research we see what is
often absent from the African scientists' report of research
findings on traditional African plant medicines, that is, an

---

[89] Ibid. It is interesting to note that traditional societies in Akwa Ibom and Cross River states, have had systems of local government organized as a federation of independent towns and villages with a common council presided over by one by one representative, presumably in rotation. And systems like it were in existence for more than 500 years before European contact. It is regrettable that in the search for effective systems of governance the Nigerian elite have never investigated ancient local systems of this type as models; the African elite has been overwhelmed by the idea that European institutions are superior to African traditional institutions.

attempt to capture the cultural background to the use of the
plant in question, as though the background details are
irrelevant or we are too embarrassed to describe the details
of "primitive" practice!

Fraser showed that the crude extract of esere bean
possessed, what in pharmacology are called anti-
cholinesterase properties: The cholinergic nerves in the
mammalian body continuously manufacture and release the
neurotransmitter substance called acetylcholine which
keeps the innervated muscles in tone and forceful
contraction when necessary. For the cholinergic system to
function properly, acetylcholine must be rapidly removed
from its site of action, as soon as it has done its work, by
the enzyme acetylcholinesterase. The esere bean contains
the alkaloid, physostigmine which blocks the
acetylcholinesterase enzyme and acetylcholine therefore
accu-mulates at nerve endings all over the body. The esere
bean in large amounts can kill a person by its anti-
cholinesterase activity, the cause of death being the
widespread action of acetylcholine in different parts of the
body—the heart, lungs, gastrointestinal tract, etc. The
manifestations of esere bean as observed in ordeal trials
and described in detail by Fraser, are clearly due to anti-
cholinesterase poisoning.

But when given in precisely measured doses, just
enough to incapacitate, the enzyme, this same action of the
poison has been found to be useful in the treatment of a
variety of diseases, for example the eye disease called
glaucoma, which can lead to blindness, and many other
serious diseases of man. The pure alkaloid, physostigmine
also known by its other name, eserine, derived from esere,
the Efik/Ibibio name for the bean, was isolated in 1865 and
structural elucidation and synthesis achieved in 1925.

Esere is, arguably, Nigeria's most important contribution to the development of modern medicine. The original obser-vations of the pharmacological action of the esere bean in human beings which eventually led to the discovery of the principal alkaloid, eserine, were made by the Efik/Ibibio people. The availability of eserine enabled the debate on neurotransmission to be settled in favour of chemical transmission, i.e., in favour of the theory that the transmission of impulse from nerve to nerve and from nerve to an innervated organ, is by means of chemical substances, a critically important principle in pharmacology and drug therapy and neurological sciences in general.

The molecule of eserine contains two tertiary nitrogen atoms. This means that eserine can cross the blood-brain barrier after oral ingestion, it can enter the brain. The blood-brain barrier is a system of capillary blood vessels that filters out potentially neurotoxic molecules from entering the brain. Studies have shown that eserine has both central (brain) and peripheral nervous system effects. An important brain effect is stimulation of the vomiting centre, whereas the effect of excessive acetylcholine accumulation in the peripheral nervous system is deadly: It slows the heart, causes copious salivation and bronchial secretions, diarrhoea, bronchospasm, cardio-vascular collapse and death.

How does the esere bean work in witchcraft detection?

Physostigmine has been studied extensively for more than 100 hundred years and a great deal is known about how it works in the body. But the question of whether the assumed capacity of the esere bean to detect witchcraft (the innocent person vomits the poison and survives, the guilty collapses and dies), can have a rational scientific explanation, has never been seriously addressed.

Does the use of esere in witchcraft detection make sense with what we know of the pharmacological actions of the main constituent of the bean, physostigmine? The question has never been asked almost certainly because the witchcraft belief and the witchcraft ordeal testing have always been thought of as a superstitious mumbo-jumbo, not suitable subjects for scientific investigation. If we were to put aside prejudice and negative propaganda regarding African traditional institutions and belief systems, we could enquire seriously into the intriguing possibility that through experience and knowledge of human nature, the people discovered that the esere bean could distinguish someone guilty of witchcraft from the innocent in an appropriately conducted ordeal trial. The fact that ancient Efik/Ibibio thinkers did not see the need to offer an explanation of how the bean worked, does not necessarily mean that the test did not have a rational experiential basis. After all, the ancient Chinese healers who first employed acupuncture as a medical procedure almost certainly did not know that peripheral nerves, when titillated by a needle, released endorphin (an endogenous painkiller). This mechanism which is now used to explain the beneficial effects of acupuncture is a modern interpretation of an ancient Chinese art in the light of biomedical discoveries made in the last three to four decades.

The answer to whether the esere bean could have distinguished between the guilty and the innocent in witchcraft detection trials, must be sought in the milieu of African culture and traditional beliefs, where, as discussed earlier, in the absence of law enforcement mechanisms, the need for strict adherence to society's moral laws was considered crucial for social harmony and survival of small kinship groups. In these circumstances, thoughts about witchcraft (whether one possessed it or not) must have been something that existed in the consciousness of the acculturated African most of the time.[90]

Considering all that we know of the pharmacological actions of physostigmine, we can speculate on how a combination of a sense of guilt (attack of conscience), or certainty of innocence (clear conscience) in the mind of the accused person on the one hand, and the absorption and distribution characteristics (the pharmacokinetics) of physostig-mine on the other, could have acted to give the ordeal trial consistency and validity in the culture where it operated.

Why the innocent vomited and survived and the guilty died has no direct empirical proof, but I offer it because it is a scientifically interesting idea that can be tested experimentally. Fear in the accused person who felt guilty could lead to a comparatively slow rate of absorption of the poison from the gastrointestinal tract, whereupon the peripheral deadly effect of esere bean would predominate. We know that in fright and anxiety there is a sympathetic nervous system-driven constriction of the splanchnic blood vessels (these are the blood vessels supplying the GIT) which means that under such conditions, there is a reduced blood flow to the gastrointestinal tract. In the person with certainty of innocence on the other hand, there is no fear-mediated constriction of splanchnic blood vessels. Therefore there would be a relatively rapid absorption of the poison into the bloodstream, whereupon central

---

[90] For references on this point see M.B. Ogunniyi, Traditional African culture and modern science, in: Nigeria since Independence: the first 25 years, vol VII, Peter Ekeh and Garba Asiwaju, editors (Ibadan, Heineman Educational Books, 1989) p. 212.

nervous system effects, including stimulation of the vomiting centre, would be the dominant effect of esere bean. There is evidence that eserine crosses the blood-brain barrier in the brain; it is known to have a variety of pharmacological actions.

Furthermore, we have to bear in mind that there is no objective mark by which a witch/wizard can be identified. There is no consensus even among believers that a witch/wizard knows for certain that she/he is one. Among the Azande where Professor Evans-Pritchard investigated this point, he concluded that the person carrying a 'witchcraft substance' might not know that he is carrying it.[91]

Therefore when an acculturated person is brought to the ordeal trial, in an emotionally charged atmosphere, a critical determinant of the outcome of taking the poison is the person's state of mind. A person who is bearing a grudge, envy or hatred against the supposed bewitched victim, may, at the point of taking the ordeal poison, pause to wonder if these emotions are what constitute witchcraft. Or, if the person knows for sure that he is guilty as charged, he would be gripped by fear knowing the power of esere bean to kill a witch. In such persons who approach the trial in a state of confusion, doubt, guilt, hesitation and fear, the poison would act in accordance with the physiological distribution of blood flow described above.

On the other hand, the innocent person who knows that she/he does not harbour witchcraft or hatred, envy, etc, would take the poison without fear or anxiety thereby favouring a rapid absorption of the poison and hence a dominant central nervous system action of the poison.

---

[91] E. Gilles, E. E. Evans-Pritchard. Witchcraft, Oracles, and Magic among the Azande (Oxford, Clarendon Press, 1976), p. 42.

It is most unlikely that the Ibibio/Efik who discovered etu esere considered the possibility of such a mechanism by which the poison exercised its power, but they understood human nature. Such a mechanism would explain why the witchcraft belief could have acted as a deterrence against antisocial behaviour or against harbouring negative emotions.

How eserine assisted in confirming the identity of "vagusstoff" and winning the Nobel Prize for physiology or medicine

It was not only the scientists of Edinburgh who gained honours from the study of esere bean, eserine was crucial to the important research of the British physiologist Sir Henry Dale and the German pharmacologist Otto Loewi, whose work eventually led to the discovery of acetylcholine as the neurotransmitter in cholinergic nerves.

At the turn of the 20th century, there were two dominant theories to explain how the impulse generated in a nerve is transmitted to another nerve or from the nerve to the organ that responds when the nerve is stimulated. The question was, what causes the heartbeat to slow down when the vagus nerve is stimulated or the skeletal muscle to contract forcefully when the motor nerve supplying it is stimulated? One theory was that the electrical impulse generated in the nerve 'jumped' across the junction between the nerve and the heart or skeletal muscle cells. It was this electrical impulse, the proponents of this theory maintained, that depolarized the heart muscle and caused the heart to beat more slowly or the skeletal muscle to contract.

The other theory was that the electrical impulse on reaching the nerve ending caused the latter to release a chemical substance which crossed the junction to act on receptors on heart muscle cells to slow the heart down. This latter theory which became known as the 'neurohumoral theory of nerve transmission' was greatly advanced by Otto Loewi's experiments on isolated frog hearts. Loewi was a German pharmacologist who was a strong advocate of the neurohumoral theory. The story was that Loewi had been thinking about an experiment to demonstrate his idea for nearly a decade; then one night the right experiment came to him in a dream. He woke up and wrote down the revelation and went back to sleep. In the morning he found he could not read his writing where he scribbled the experiment! Fortunately for science and humanity, the dream obligingly returned the following night! This time Otto Loewi set off immediately to the laboratory at 3.00 a.m. to put up the experiment![92]

He perfused two frog hearts in series (the physiological salt solution emerging from one heart then perfused a second heart whose vagus nerve had been cut); he then stimulated the vagus nerve to the first ('donor') heart whose beat immediately slowed down, followed a few moments later by the slowing of the 'recipient' (second) heart; something (vagusstoff) had been released from the vagus nerve of the donor's heart which slowed the two hearts, Otto Loewi concluded. But what was vagusstoff?

At about the same time, Dale was experimenting with anaesthetized cats, and finding that the stimulation of the vagus nerve slowed cats' hearts and lowered the blood pressure. The chemical substance, acetylcholine which Dale and Barger had synthesized, caused similar effects to those of vagus stimulation, when injected into the cat's

---

[92] Paraphrased from H.P. Rang, M.M. Dale & J.M. Ritter, Pharmacology 4th ed.(Edinburgh,Churchill Livingstone,1999) p. 95.

vein. Both effects were transient. Dale recognized that acetylcholine being an ester would be hydrolysed very rapidly by esterase enzymes present in plasma, which would account for the transient action of injected acetylcholine. Dale therefore suspected that the substance released by the vagus nerve (Loewi's vagusstoff) might also be an ester like acetylcholine.

All was revealed by eserine which had by now become available; the synthesis of eserine had been achieved in 1925. By inhibiting acetyl-cholinesterase enzyme thereby preserving the acetylcholine released when the vagus nerve was stimulated, eserine potentiated the effect of vagal stimulation and acetylcholine injection. This was the crucial evidence which enabled Dale and Loewi to reach the final conclusion that acetylcholine is the neurotransmitter mediating the effect of the vagus nerve stimulation. This was subsequently confirmed at other parasympathetic and motor nerves and direct identification of acetylcholine in perfusates.

Dale and Loewi shared the 1936 Nobel Prize for physiology or medicine "for their discoveries relating to the chemical transmission of nerve impulses".[93] The conclusive evidence in support of the theory of neurohumoral trans-mission, one of the most important principles in medicine, could not have been secured, when it was achieved, without eserine. The importance of this discovery can be appreciated if we bear in mind that the human body functions as it does through a coordinated action of a massive network of different nerves and neurons operating in unison in different parts of the body, and the mediators

---

[93] W.F. Bynum, An Early History of the British Pharmacological Society, (London: British Pharmacological Society, 1981) p. 9.

of this complex coordinated action are neurotransmitters, one of them being acetylcholine.

Efik/Ibibio were not accorded intellectual property rights
Let me point out that apart from the occasional reference to the Efik/Ibibio as the first people to use esere bean as ordeal poison in witchcraft detection, there is no recognition of the huge significance of their original discovery and clinical demonstration of esere bean effects in human beings, in the vast literature on Calabar bean. Quite clearly, before arriving at the point when the Efik/Ibibio ancients and their communities could conclude that esere bean was a consistently reliable mechanism for discriminating between the guilty and the innocent, in witchcraft detection, there must have been a long process of trial and error. In a sense, the use of the esere bean in public ordeal witchcraft trials by the Efik/Ibibio people was among the earliest experience of controlled clinical trials. It is a reflection of the extent to which European intelligentsia unhesitatingly disregarded the possibility of rational thought in what Africans did that the question of how these people came to use a poison in this complex way never arose.

We note that (i) nowhere in the records is credit given to the Ibibio/Efik ancients for their original discovery of esere bean and their demonstration of its pharmacological properties in open ordeal witchcraft trials, which eventually provoked scientific investigation of the poison. (ii) Eserine and newer synthetic drugs based on its structure, e.g., neostigmine, have been used worldwide for decades in the treatment of glaucoma, certain disorders of the urinary and gastrointestinal tracts, muscular dystrophy, Alzheimer's disease and various disease conditions where the need to increase the concentration of acetylcholine is a clinical imperative. No portion of the huge profits made from the sales of these drugs ever came to Ibibio/Efik land. The people were denied their intellectual property rights.

It was presumed then and now by 'bio-prospectors' (biomedical scientists prospecting for drugs from traditional biological sources) that indigenous traditional African knowledge is not knowledge as such as it is known in the West, since it was assumed not to be empirically derived, and it was not associated with an individual's name holding a patent! The thinking was that ancient Africans knew whatever they knew by instinct, not through rational thought that came from experience and observation.

Let me conclude by emphasizing the point that although eserine has many uses in modern medicine as a drug, the indigenous people who discovered esere bean and its "pharmacological properties" and used it in witchcraft ordeal trials never used it as a therapy for healing purposes. This fact is consistent with my proposition that the repertoire of traditional herbal remedies tended to exclude poisonous plants.

The other important point to draw out of the story of the esere bean, is that educated Africans, in their anxiety to make 'progress' in a European-dominated world, have been unwilling to take the initiative to explore traditional African knowledge systems, even when its vast possibilities are staring us in the face. In this regard, we can say it was fortunate that Fraser (1863) and other Europeans carried out a detailed study of esere bean (1925) over 100 years ago, if they did not, medical science would have been poorer for it. Left to Nigerian medical scientists, that study would probably not have been done. Even though esere bean research has been going on for one-hundred years or more, there remains a formidable esere bean phytochemical arsenal of chemical entities of medicinal value waiting to be investigated.

Then there is the intriguing question of the possible mechanism by which esere bean could have discriminated between the guilty and the innocent in witchcraft detection. A proper study of this phenomenon could open up a whole range of interesting possibilities for a drug like physostigmine and the way emotion affects drug action. Furthermore, there are numerous other witchcraft ordeal poisonous plants that are widely known in other parts of Nigeria which have not been scientifically investigated, and which may yield molecules with selective toxicity suitable for development into drugs for use in modern medicine.

The fact of the matter is that witchcraft is not a subject to which Nigerian scientists are attracted, either because of fear of witchcraft or the fact that the belief in the doctrine was denigrated in early European writings as a product of ignorance and superstition. That is why today, although witchcraft is currently believed to wreak havoc in many Nigerian communities, Nigerian scientists, social scientists, anthro-pologists and philosophers have not embraced it as a serious and worthy subject of study, which would help to tame the belief. In our present pentecostal religious climate it is hard to imagine a Nigerian scientist giving a testimony before his/her church congregation that his special research interest is witchcraft!

Chapter 10

From Poison to Drug: Examples of dramatic discoveries in Europe

The development of the important drug physostigmine from what was known in traditional Efik/Ibibio society as an ordeal poison is not exceptional in the history of medicine. In this chapter I describe some other well known examples of drugs from poisons in Europe, partly because their stories are interesting and also to demonstrate that such experience was widespread; and to further underscore two points that are relevant to the present discussion of traditional African medicine theory: First, none of the drugs to be described was used in traditional European medicine, at the very least, not for the treatment of the disease for which the drug is now famous in modern medicine. Second, the desperate need to standardize the poisonous plant digitalis, so that it could be used safely in the treatment of dropsy, was a critical driving force in the development of bioassay, a development that led to the emergence of precision measurements which eventually enabled poisonous substances to be routinely used in modern medicine as drugs.

Digitalis

Digitalis purpurea (its other evocative names in English are: Witches Clove, Foxglove, Deadman's Thimbles and Blood Fingers). This plant can be found throughout Europe. According to mythology the mottled marks on the flowers were put there by the gods to warn of the dangerously poisonous juices secreted by the plant. The use of the foxglove by ancient European herbalists, bears no relationship to the use today of products derived from it. They are the most important drugs in the treatment of cardiac disease.

Welsh traditional physicians of the 13th century used foxglove in the treatment of fresh wounds, sores and ulcers, bruises and boils as external medication only, it being considered too poisonous for internal use. The crude drug was included in the London Pharmacopoeia of 1650.

More than 100 years later, we are told, a Shropshire woman drew Sir William Withering's attention to the possible usefulness of foxglove in the treatment of dropsy (oedema associated with congestive heart failure) and digitalis leaf eventually became official in the British Pharmacopoeia (B.P.) for many years, but it is the glycosides extracted from the leaf digoxin, digitoxin that are now widely used in the treatment of congestive heart failure.

It is interesting to note that the digitalis leaf was used in European traditional medicine for various purposes for over 500 years before its cardiac properties for which it is famous today, were isolated.

In the right dose, digitalis caused dramatic improvement in cardiac function and was effective in the treatment of dropsy as it increased cardiac output and urine production with subsequent reduction in oedema of the extremities. But if only slightly higher doses were given, it was fatally toxic due to its action on the heart. Digitalis is thus said to have a narrow margin of safety or low therapeutic index, that is to say, the difference between the dose that cures and the dose that kills, is small, and because the digitalis leaf from different sources varied greatly in potency, it became necessary to standardize the crude drug for maximum therapeutic benefit.

As stated earlier, a poisonous substance can only be a useful drug when it can be given in precise quantities. The need to standardize the digitalis leaf therefore became a critical impetus for the development of a reproducible method for the biological assay (the quantitative determination of a drug by measurement of its biological activity) of digitalis leaf from different sources. The availability of a reproducible biological assay method enabled digitalis leaf to be widely usable in medicine. Bioassay methods were also soon developed for the standardization of other crude natural product medicines. The official standard assay of Tincture of Digitalis Leaf B.P. depended on the volume of the tincture (the alcoholic extract of digitalis leaf) prepared according to specified procedures that would, on infusion, cause cessation of the heartbeat in an anaesthetized guinea pig. This was a crude method of standardization, but it served the purpose of making a useful and life-saving drug out of an otherwise poisonous substance. The availability of pure digitalis glycosides and precision technology, have rendered the old methods of assay obsolete.

These new advances do not detract from the historical importance of early bioassay methods in the development of drugs. Pharmacologists take pride in this. They say that pharmacology as a discipline has borrowed many of its ideas and methods from other disciplines—physiology, biochemistry, molecular biology, physics, chemistry, genetics, etc, and applied them to drug development, but pharmacology has one defining method of its own, namely, bioassay. Bioassay was the foundation of modern pharmacology and drug development.

Dicoumarol

In the winter of 1921 to 1922 veterinarians in the Province of Alberta, Canada reported a new disease called 'sweet clover disease' that killed large numbers of cattle that had eaten, what turned out to be, badly stored and spoiled clover. The disease was characterized by massive bleeding. The haemorrhage was caused by a poison in the spoilt clover which the vets called melilotoxin. Crude extracts of spoilt clover successfully reproduced sweet clover disease in laboratory rabbits, but it took scientists in North America and Europe another 20 years for the "agent of death" bishydroxycoumarin or dicoumarol to be isolated and chemically identified.

Dicoumarol is an anticoagulant. It was the first substance known to inhibit the production of prothrombin in the liver. The formation of prothrombin is a critical step in the cascade of reactions leading to the clotting of blood. Dicoumarol and its synthetic derivatives have become an important class of drugs known as anticoagulants now widely used in modern medicine in surgery, heart disease, management of stroke, etc. Not only that, the introduction of dicoumarol has increased the understanding of the complex mechanisms involved in blood clotting.

Ergot alkaloids

Claviceps purpura or ergot is a fungus of the genus Ulstilago that grows on rye and other grains. The contamination of edible grain by this poisonous parasite caused death and destruction periodically for many centuries in different parts of Europe. The affliction was characterized by gangrene of the legs, hands and arms. In severe cases of ergot poisoning, "the tissue becomes dry and black and the mummified limbs separate off without loss of blood". The disease was referred to as St. Anthony's fire. Those who managed to visit the shrine of St. Anthony recovered from the illness, explained cynically as being due to the fact that the pilgrims had refrained from eating contaminated bread during their sojourn at the shrine!

From about 1670, reports on ergot began to appear in medical journals, and once it was recognized that the fungus contained the poison that caused ergot poisoning and so much havoc, European scientists among them Barger, a close associate of Sir Henry Dale (see the esere bean chapter 9), set out to identify the chemical entities in ergot which turned out to be a library of numerous pharmacologically active agents including several alkaloids, one of them being the famous hallucinogen, lysergic acid diethylamide (LSD), methysergide and ergotamine (used in the treatment of migraine), ergometrine (used in obstetrics in the treatment of postpartum haemorrhage) and many more.

Searching for drugs in African plants of medical interest

One huge area of interest in TAM is the development of modern drugs from African plants of medicinal interest. In the past such a search was guided by traditional healers' claims of the effectiveness of certain plants in the treatment of diseases, and anecdotes of that sort. Such research was based on the assumptions that the aims of traditional healers' use of plant remedies were the same as those of drugs in modern medicine. We have seen that this is not so.

African plants are a huge potential source of medicine, but to be successful in translating that potential into reality, the plants to be investigated must be chosen with care and a well considered protocol. The number of species of higher plants on planet earth is estimated to be between 370 000 and 500 000. All higher plants elaborate secondary chemical metabolites that are entities of potential therapeutic interest. Therefore, a careful consideration of the criteria for selecting a plant for phytotherapeutic investigation is probably as important an exercise as the investigation itself. For this reason several factors that should guide plant selection have been described in previous publications.[94] With regard to the search for drugs in African plants in particular, and the discussions so far concerning the use of herbal medicines in TAM, it may help to elaborate on the following two potential sources of drugs:

i. Poisonous plants

As already suggested, the search for drugs with high selective toxicity in African plants, is more likely to succeed if we focus our attention on poisonous plants (arrow poisons, ordeal poisons, fish poisons, etc) that are known by indigenous people who usually avoid such plants as therapy, than on plants used regularly by them for the treatment of disease.

This suggestion turns the basis of our conventional approaches to the search for drugs in TAM remedies on its head. The idea that we should turn to poisonous plants in search of drugs, instead of the conventional approach in which the search is based on traditional healers' claims of effectiveness of particular plants, is not a frivolous suggestion, rather it logically arises from TAM theory and from historical reality. As is well known, many drugs in use in modern medicine today were extracted from plants. What is not usually mentioned in the same breath is that most of such drugs were extracted from well

---

[94]E.M. Williamson, D.T. Okpako and Fred Evans, Pharmacological Methods in Phytotherapy Research (John Wiley & Sons, New York, 1996) pp. 5-7.

known poisonous plants. Some important examples of such plants have been described above in the two preceding chapters.

We can add a few more for emphasis: picrotoxin, a barbiturate overdose antidote, was extracted from Anamirta cocculus, known in many parts of the world as fish poison; atropine and analogues derived from it, used widely in modern drug therapy, was originally extracted from Datura strammonium, which is recognized in traditional communities as a poisonous plant all over West Africa; ouabain— used for treating congestive heart failure—was extracted from gratus Strophanthus , known in East and Central Africa as arrow poison. Thus, it is a fact that communities in Africa know

poisonous plants even though they do not, as a rule, use them as medicine. The reasons why this is so have already been extensively discussed, but historical experience indicates that such plants are a potential source of molecules that can be developed as drugs for use in modern medicine.

ii. Plants commonly used in the treatment of minor
    ailments as a source of drugs

The other source which research can exploit as a source of drugs for use in modern medicine, are the plants commonly used by indigenous African people to treat common ailments such as fever, aches and pains, bleeding, stomach upset, etc. The principles underlying the treatment of minor ailments in TAM, is the subject matter in Part 3 of the book. It goes without saying that the search for drugs for use in modern medicine can also benefit from the vast knowledge of plant remedies used in the treatment of common/minor ailments among indigenous populations.

It may seem like a contradiction to suggest that traditional African herbal remedies used in the treatment of common ailments can be a source of drugs in view of my deposition earlier that poisonous plants should be the focus of the search for drugs of the type commonly used in modern medicine. It can be argued that the distinction between drugs in modern medicine and herbal medicines in TAM based on the grounds that modern drugs are selectively toxic poisons, whereas herbal medicines are not, is an oversimplification of a complex issue; even the commonly used herbal remedies also possess chemical entities that are selectively toxic to the cause of the minor ailments they are used to treat. For example, research results worldwide show that a common pharmacological property of extracts of commonly used traditional herbal remedies is anti-inflammatory activity. The inflammation phenomenon involves many reaction steps that are catalysed by different enzymes, for example, cyclooxygenases, lipoxegenases; nitric oxide synthase e.t.c., and, as can be seen the review by Peter Akah and Sylvester Nworu,[95] herbal medicines contain chemical entities that can selectively inhibit these different enzymes to bring relief from minor ailments. Examples of anti-inflammatory, antioxidants, immuno-stimulatory chemical groups found in herbal remedies and indeed in

---

[95] See appendix 2, pages 329-358.

different foods and red wine, are flavonoids such as kaempferol and quercetin; flavones and benzoquinones; phenolic compounds, triterpenes, sesquiterpene lactones etc, that can block many aspects of the inflammation response.

Therefore, traditional herbal remedies and drugs are alike in selectively inhibiting a biological target to bring about relief. In other words, the definition that "all (chemical) substances are poisons; there is none which is not a poison, the right dose differentiates a poison from a remedy", applies to herbal remedies as well as to modern drugs. A point well taken!

However, I argue that there is no contradiction in suggesting that drugs for use in modern medicine can be developed from poisonous plants and from herbal remedies used in the treatment of common ailments on the grounds that the drugs developed from the two sources will be different, analogical to modern medicine's two categories of drugs:

   i.   those drugs that can be used only on a prescription from a qualified physician called, prescription only medicines (POM), and

   ii.   those medicines that can be bought over the counter without a prescription called (OTC) medicines.

POM drugs are those that can be described as poisons deployed for therapeutic purposes, whose type is more likely to be discovered in poisonous African plants. A POM drug is prescribed for a clearly diagnosed disease, and must be used strictly according to a specified dose schedule as described fully in chapter 12 on the Dose of Medicine (p.209). Over-the- counter drugs are not subject to the strict control described for POM, they are available for self-diagnosed ailments without a doctor's prescription. Herbal remedies, as has been shown, derive from the pharmacopoeia of non poisonous plants. They have the attributes of drugs in the category of OTC medicines. They can be taken without divination or incantations, guided only by the individual's previous experience of the usefulness of the remedy.

The main ground for drawing a distinction between POM and OTC drugs is safety. Knowing that all drugs have unwanted side effects, a critical determinant of the usefulness of a drug in modern medicine is its margin of safety, technically defined as the therapeutic index which is roughly the ratio of the dose of the drug that will cause harm or kill the patient, to the dose that will cure the patient Prescription-only-drugs have narrow margins of safety, that is, the difference between toxic and therapeutic doses is small, hence the need to strictly control their use; whereas the margins are wider for OTC drugs. For traditional African herbal remedies the margins of safety are unknown, but can be assumed to be large for reasons alluded to already.

The important question that arises when contemplating the development of medicines from traditional African herbal remedies that can be used in modern medicine is this: Should the products be used much as they are in TAM or should research proceed to the isolation and identification of individual chemical entities in the remedy, with a view to the production of drugs. Perhaps the aim should be a combination of both approaches. The medicine produced as a herbal remedy would be used in TAM, but a phytochemical analysis would enable each plant to be standardized in terms of its most active anti-inflammatory chemical entity. This is the sort of issue that should be a major concern of a centre devoted to the study of inflammation and malaria.

Chapter 11

Speculations on the Origins of the Pharmacopoeia of Plant Remedies in Traditional African Medicine

I n virtually all African communities the people know plants that are commonly used to treat minor ailments, and each traditional healer in the community has his/her own repertoire of plant remedies. The question is how did indigenous people arrive at the knowledge of plants that can be used routinely for the treatment of diseases frequently experienced in their communities?

It would seem that throughout human history, indigenous populations autochthonously came to the knowledge of important plant remedies for the treatment of the diseases that afflicted them most frequently. For example, African populations who were in contact with the Anopheles mosquito and suffered frequent bouts of fever (malaria) were also in the forefront in the development of anti-fever plant remedies that are known widely in these communities. I have also pointed out that in African medicine, a likely criterion for including a plant in the repertoire of remedies was that the plant was not overtly poisonous; in other words, indigenous people may have deliberately excluded poisonous plants from their pharmacopoeia of remedies. However, in addition to those sorts of pre-scientific instinctive ways of knowing critically important plant remedies, there are some other interesting ideas/theories about how indigenous African communities discovered medicinal plants. These theories are examined briefly below.

i.   Trial and error theory

The idea behind this theory is that through a process of trial and error, people over evolutionary time, selected those plants that were found to be therapeutically beneficial in treating particular diseases.[96] This theory essentially attributes the healing power of plant remedies to the specific pharmacological action of their chemical constituents, similar to drugs in modern medicine. This implies that if a traditional healer claims that a certain plant is useful in the treatment of, say, diabetes, we must assume that through a process of trial and error, the healer or community of healers selected that particular plant for its efficacy in the treatment of diabetes, and must possess anti-diabetic principles. This has been used as a guiding principle for the selection of African plants to be investigated in search of drugs.

---

[96] E.J. Shellard, The significance of research into medicinal plants. In: A. Sofowora, editor, African Medicinal Plants. Proceedings, Pan African Conference on Research into Medicinal Plants, at the University of Ife, Ile-Ife in April 1974. (University of Ife Press, Ile-Ife, Nigeria 1979).

It is easy to see why this idea appeals to the biomedical scientist. Many modern drugs have in fact been developed through a process of trial and error. Based on the theory that chemical structures can somehow predict pharmacological activity (the structure-action relationship principle), the synthetic organic chemist makes a large number of compounds from a template, and through screening, evaluation and clinical trials, a few promising compounds are selected for further development. Other compounds that do not pass the initial screen are rejected. During the Vietnam War, for example, when American forces were deployed in large numbers in malaria endemic terrains, Walter Reed Army Hospital scientists tested more than 300,000 chloroquine-like compounds for anti-malaria activity of which one compound, mefloquine came through after trials that spanned more than ten years, and the expenditure of tens of millions of American dollars. Mefloquine is toxic, but by the time it became available for general use, the Vietnam War was over and its major beneficiaries were Africans and other people living in malaria endemic parts of the world where the toxicity/benefit ratio was considered acceptable.

Another example is the anti-ulcer drug tagamet, developed by James Black and his team at the Smyth, Klein and French pharmaceutical laboratory. The team started with the idea that a drug that would cure ulcer must contain a molecule that specifically blocked histamine H2-receptors, and that such a molecule was likely to be a modified structure of histamine itself. The theory was that histamine, acting at H2-receptor as agonist was the cause of the ulcer, by stimulating the production of excessive hydrochloric acid. Therefore, the way to stop this kind of ulcer was to find a specific histamine H2-receptor antagonist. Black's synthetic chemists proceeded to make numerous derivatives of the histamine molecule which were subjected to anti-ulcer screens, out of which cimetidine (tagamet) emerged as a suitable drug. These are target-directed trial and error approaches based on sound scientific principles, but trial and error just the same.

These examples, by the way, illustrate the great difficulties inherent in trial and error methods even when the new compounds to be tried were synthesized using predictable template molecules. In the case of mefloquine the template molecule was the powerful anti-malaria drug chloroquine, and in the case of tagamet, the template was the well known H2-receptor agonist molecule, histamine.

Did the plants used as remedies in TAM evolve from any sort of therapeutic trial? I think not. It does not help the validation of TAM to insist that its remedies arose from a retrospective reasoning. What is most likely is that if a plant was deadly poisonous on ingestion, it would over time become excluded from the treatment regimen of traditional healers, and the word would go round about that particular property of the plant. This, of course, is a form of trial and error, but it is distinctively different from 'trial' for a specific therapeutic activity implied by the theory. The trial and error hypothesis implies that traditional African healers had detailed knowledge of plants and could distinguish between related species. It also implies that the practice of TAM involved detailed knowledge of classes of diseases, each with a specific herbal treatment. This was most probably not the case; attributing to African medicine what we know now in modern medicine, that there are different classes of disease, and that there are different species of plants that can be used to treat those diseases, is a fallacious retrospective reasoning. There is little evidence to support the view that such detailed classification ever formed the basis of plant selection for the treatment of disease in TAM. Traditional medicine practitioners when dealing with serious illness are more concerned with "illness" rather than with the specific diseases that gave rise to the illness.

To take one example, the Ughievwen word for cough, akpanran, is the identification term for all illnesses in which cough is a manifestation, e.g., tuberculosis, asthma, bronchitis or pneumonia; they are all akpanran of different grades of severity. The traditional healer may use one plant remedy for bronchitis and asthma. His choice of plant remedy for bronchitis would therefore not be a good guide in the search for compounds with a potential for the treatment of asthma.

Furthermore, although traditional African societies knew a great deal about plants in their immediate surroundings, it is doubtful whether this knowledge was deep and detailed enough to sustain trial and error of plants for the treatment of specific diseases. Isawumi has described a Yoruba system of naming plants and concluded that "the problem of nomenclature is one reason that prevents traditional medicine from realizing its full potential".[97] In Yoruba plant nomenclature, "two plants sharing a common name . . . may belong to, not only different genera but even to different families; for example, ewuro ijebu (Ijebu bitter leaf, Solanum eritum, Fam. Solanaceae) and ewuro odo (riverine bitter leaf, Striuchium sparagnophora, Fam. Compositae)." In chemical composition and therefore pharmacological profile, these two plants are completely different even though they are both known as ewuro in the Yoruba language.

This is not to deny that in general, indigenous populations have intimate knowledge of the local vegetation, including knowledge of trees believed to have healing powers. The Iroko tree (Chlorophora excelsa), for example, is regarded as sacred in many communities in Nigeria. Sacrificial offerings are frequently found at its base. Images of household gods and clan deities are carved from the iroko wood. Apart from the fact that iroko wood is first class quality timber, it is believed that images carved from the wood and medicines made from its bark, have special spiritual potencies.

Another example is the tree known to Edo people as Akuobisi (Akuobaka aubreville). This tree is treated with awe and reverence. It is believed that the tree is inhabited by a fiery spirit with many myths about its power. The following paraphrased account was given to me by the famous Edo forester, the late Chief A.M. Oseni, one time

---

[97] M. Isawumi, Yoruba system of plant nomenclature and its implications in traditional medicine. Nigerian Field 1990 (55): 165-171.

Director of Forestry of the Federal Republic of Nigeria:

> On approaching it the Edo address it as
> "akuobisi, non ogieran" meaning 'akuobisi,
> the king of trees'. The bark must be removed
> with caution, and not at sunrise or sunset,
> when the spirit of akuobisi is going out or
> coming in. If you wish to take the bark, the
> spirit of akuobisi must be appeased with
> offerings of kola nuts, white chalk, cooked
> yam and palm oil before taking the bark of
> the tree. Under no circumstances must a
> machete or other sharp metal instruments be
> used on akuobisi, only a piece of wood must
> be used to remove a piece of medicinal bark.
> You must approach akuobisi stark naked,
> and after obtaining the required piece of
> bark, the healer must run away from the tree
> and put on his clothes as fast as he can. This
> is in case akuobisi is not satisfied with the
> offered sacrifice and the spirit comes after
> the healer, he would not recognize him now
> fully clothed. The fact that nothing
> whatsoever grows under its canopy is
> believed to due to the power of the spirit in
> akuobisi. [98]

But, there is also a lack of consistency between
traditional healers or even by the same healer, in the use

---

[98] The conservation significance of this myth is obvious. How much bark can you
remove using a piece of wood? Only the determined healer would have taken the
trouble to go to Akuobisi! Trees with this kind of mythical reputation, grew and
survived for centuries, before the advent of European pressure in Africa.

of plants with respect to the specific diseases or conditions for which the plant is used. The same plant may be used for illnesses for which opposite pathological principles are at play. For example, the plant Zizyphus mauritania is claimed by a set of Yoruba traditional healers to be effective in the treatment of constipation and by another set for the treatment of dysentery. This prompted Professor Shellard[99] to wonder, "Can it really be effective in both?"

The plant Crotolaria retusa (koropo) is a common ingredient in medicines used by traditional healers in the Ibadan metropolis. Maclean interviewed 100 herbalists in the area to ascertain which diseases they used koropo to treat.

> It was used variously as an analgesic, for dysentery, an aid to conception (it was thought to help to retain sperm in the vagina) and to induce labour. Some herbalists claimed that the plant could aid memory in school children and that koropo "would persuade an abiku child to stay... induce a divorced wife to return to her husband, guard a house and its occupants against dangerous medicine . . . and assist in the arrest of evildoers and lunatics. [100]

---

[99] Ibid, see footnote 99.

[100] Una Maclean, Choices of treatment among the Yoruba, in: Culture and Curing, Perspectives on traditional medical beliefs and practices P. Morley and R. Willis, editors (London, Peter Owen Ltd, 1978) p. 84.

It is most unlikely that koropo evolved for use in these different conditions following processes of trial and error. The perception among African traditional healers that plants have extraordinary powers is evident from the array of magical claims made for koropo above, but it is doubtful whether it was ever tried and found to be capable of "inducing a divorced wife to return to her husband".

ii. Animal lead hypothesis and the Gombe chimpanzee's medicine chest

Another view of how plant remedies evolved in African medicine is what might be called the "the animal lead" hypothesis. This proposes that medicinal plants were identified by man, after observing sick animals eat such plants and become well. It is difficult to see how humans, who are susceptible to quite a different range of diseases from animals (and many animal diseases are species specific), would be led to healing plants by animals; but the idea persists and I will cite two examples of how it has been expressed. According to Professor Abayomi Sofowora[101] of the Obafemi Awolowo University that kind of observation could have been made by hunters--

> When for example, a hunter shot an
> elephant, if the elephant ran away, chewed
> leaves from a specific plant, and did not die,
> it is believed that the hunter noted the plant

---

[101] Medicinal Plants and Traditional Medicine in Africa (Chichester, John Wiley and Sons Limited, 1982) p.13.

as a possible antidote for wounds or for
relieving pain.

No examples of plant remedies that were discovered by
this mechanism are given, but a later report on
chimpanzees based on the same idea in the New Scientist
[102]contains observations made by the distinguished prize-
winning primatologist Jane Goodall and anthropologist
Richard Wrangham on how the chimpanzees in the
Gombe Stream National Park in Tanzania, deliberately
ate the young leaves of the plants Aplasia pluriseta and
Aplasia rudies which the local Tongwe Africans happen
to also use as medicine for the treatment of a wide range
of ailments. The young leaves of Aplasia were, on
phytochemical analysis, found to contain a chemical
substance thiarubrine-A, which had antimicrobial and
antihelmintic (worm expelling) properties. The scientists
therefore concluded that both the Africans and the
chimpanzees use Aplasia leaves for the same medicinal
purposes, and the scientists were ---

> . . . struck by the wisdom of the chimp and
> the African peoples, who figured out,
> without the benefit of a high-tech analysis
> that the young leaves contain the potent
> chemical.

The authors do not say whether the chimps were ill
before they ate Aplasia and whether the chimps' health
improved after eating it. The only clue as to the possible
health benefit of the plant to the chimps was the

---

[102] Cathy Sears, The chimpanzee's medicine chest. New Scientist, vol. 127 (Aug. 4,
1990), pp. 42-44.

observation that the chimps' faeces contained a variety of parasites "which might prompt the chimps to seek relief by treating themselves with the appropriate plant". It is an impressive leap of imagination to conclude from the fact that chimpanzees ate aplasia leaves which happen to contain an interesting chemical entity thiarubrine, that the animals were suffering from worm infection and had deliberately selected this plant as remedy!

Let us be reminded that chimps are predominantly vegetarian and probably found young Aplasia leaves delicious! Is the presence of parasites in a chimpanzee's faeces diagnostic of illness in the animal? What if it is not? What if parasites are normal inhabitants of a chimpanzee's gut, like coliform bacteria in the human gut? And what can this unique faculty be that is possessed by chimpanzees and Tongwe Africans that enables them to identify complex chemical entities and their pharmacological properties in plants, without the benefit of high tech analysis? One senses a faint suggestion of the ancient European outmoded racist notion (not borne out in genetic data) that Africans have more in common with monkeys than with other humans!

iii. Doctrine of signatures

Another idea is the co-called doctrine of signatures credited to the 15th century Swiss physician Theophrastus von Hohen-heim (born in 1493) who promoted the idea that medicinal plants were the gifts of the gods who had endowed them with marks or symbols to indicate the part of the human body or what disease they were meant to treat.

This principle is widely recognized and applied in African therapeutic systems. For example, among the Yoruba of Western Nigeria, certain plants in the physician's remedy "seem to be included for reasons of their symbolic affinity to a disease organ".[103] Thus a Yoruba herbalist's remedy for inadequate erection 'usually includes plantains and a plant whose stem is particularly springy'. Part of a Yoruba Ijala Ode (hunters' poem) reads[104]:

> Bi mba j'ogede tan, oko mi a dide gboin
> After I have eaten roasted plantain,
> My penis will rise powerfully

The climbing plant Rauvolfia serpentina is an ingredient in snake bite remedies. Preparations made from the rhinoceros' horn are believed, in parts of Asia, to be an aphrodisiac to strengthen male erection. The demand for rhino horns is causing a decimation of the rhinoceros population in East Africa! The leaf used by one of my

---

[103] Maclean, op cit.

[104] Personal communication from Femi Fatoba, 1984.

interviewees[105] to increase the volume of the ejaculation as part of his treatment of infertility, produces a slimy secretion, similar in texture to human semen (see also page ....for the incantation that accompanies the prescription for male fertility)

Victor Turner[106]recorded the following principle in Ndembu healers' treatment of infertility:

> Trees from which bark string can be made are never used . . . to make women fertile, as these would tie up their fertility . . . the trees used have many fruits; the doctors trusted that their patients would have many children. Other trees had honey-filled flowers attractive to bees. By using them the doctors hoped to attract many children to their patients.

The following are other examples of the application of the doctrine of signatures in the selection of treatments from other parts of the world: saxifrages grow on rocks and break up stone. The plant is famously used in the treatment of stones in the gall bladder. The plant Euphrasia officinalis (eye bright) has a pupil-like spot on the flower, it has been used for centuries in Europe to "help the dimness of sight or to treat an inflamed eye".[107]

---

[105] Saradje, personal communication with a traditional healer.

[106] Drums of Affliction - A study of religious processes among the Ndemu of Zambia (London, IAP Hutchinson University for Africa, 1981)p. 61-62.

[107] B. Oliver-Bever, Medicinal Plants in Tropical West Africa. (Cambridge, Cambridge University Press, 1986) p. 5.

Throughout human history indigenous peoples' selection of plant remedies seems to have been guided by a variety of symbols, from divine revelation, such as by the Ifa oracle, or personal dreams, trial and error of some sort, or a resemblance of the plant to the problem to be treated. What is certain is that none of the plant selection modes alluded to were guided by considerations of the likely pharmacological profile of the plants' constituents. And there is no empirical evidence of a specific nature to support some of the claims, e.g., that rhinoceros' horn has male erection enhancing properties. What we can say is that the peoples' belief in the potency of the remedy contributed to its clinical benefit in synergism with whatever beneficial constituents, e.g., anti-inflammatory chemical entities which we know to be present virtually universally in plants. It is important to emphasize that a significant guiding principle was that the plant did not cause overt toxic effects.

Chapter 12

Dose of Medicine

T o successfully use potentially poisonous substances as drugs in modern medicine, it is necessary from the beginning, to strictly regulate the dose of the drug, to avoid undesirable toxic and possibly fatal side effects. How to use drugs in such a controlled way is an important part of the syllabus used in the training of the modern medical personnel who are therefore apprehensive when they find that in African medicine, plant remedies are administered without due regard to the rules of dosage. This is a common criticism of African medicine which, on this score, is considered dangerous and of doubtful validity.

Strict control of dosage in modern medicine is predicated on the theory of selective toxicity. The elementary assumption in this theory and in pharmacology in general, is that the effect of a drug is directly proportional to the amount administered. Obviously therefore, it is important to know the dose at which the action of the drug will be selective for the therapeutic target. If the quantity of drug is not strictly controlled, the drug might interact with unintended structures in the body and cause unwanted side effects, these considerations do not apply in traditional African medicine (TAM) in the management of serious illness, principally because here, the dousing of emotional tension rather than the selective poisoning of a cause is the major therapeutic objective.

Attributes of the dose of drug

Those not trained in medicine or pharmacy may not fully appreciate all that the term "dose of medicine/drug" implies. A drug is known by its many dose characteristics:

(a) Effective dose, being the dose that is sufficient to check the progress of the disease (e.g., to kill the causative agent or prevent its growth).

(b) Toxic or overdose, being the dose larger than the effective dose that may harm or kill the patient. The ratio of the toxic dose to the effective dose, called the therapeutic index (TI) describes the safety margin of the drug. Some drugs, e.g., digitalis have a low TI and must be used with great care as a slight over dose can result in a harmful effect. We can note here that because herbal remedies used in African medicine are largely non poisonous plants, these remedies would have large therapeutic indices, i.e., large safety margins. They can be taken without adherence to strict rules of dosage.

(c) The dosing interval, being the time interval (in hours) between individual doses. This is of crucial importance in modern medicine to ensure that the required effective concentration of the drug is maintained in the patient's body throughout the period of treatment. A drug's dosing interval depends on its pharmacokinetics (the elimination profile) which is different with different drugs.

(d) The dosing duration being the total period for which the drug must be taken to ensure that the disease is eliminated or brought under control. This period varies according to disease: the period is short, a few days, where the objective is to kill off an infective agent such as in malaria, bacterial or viral infection, but where the objective is to control the disease so that it does not progress to the point where it can kill the patient, for example, hypertension, diabetes or Parkinson's disease etc, the dosing duration may be for life.

As we shall see below, the pattern of use of herbal remedies in TAM differs substantially with regard to each of the four dose characteristics that are applicable to drugs in modern medicine.

Why adherence to the rules of dosage need
not apply in TAM
It would be apparent from the argument so far why strict adherence to dosage was not necessary with the use of herbal remedies in traditional medicine. We explain this by the absence of precision technology in African culture, the inherent assumptions about what causes illness in African traditional thought and the exclusion of poisonous plants from the TAM pharmacopoeia. This is

not to say that the absence of precision technology in African culture, which partly accounts for why rules of dosage do not operate in TAM, is a particular virtue; it simply emphasizes that the differences between drugs in modern medicine and herbal remedies in TAM, is a reflection of the different therapeutic objectives in the two traditions. This is illustrated by the following points, through which I draw attention to the beliefs governing the use of plant remedies in TAM and why it is inappropriate to expect this to correspond to drug use in modern medicine.

(1) In the management of serious illness in TAM, herbal medicines can be tied in a cloth/leather pouch and worn as a bracelet, a necklace, an amulet, a waistband or placed under the pillow or sleeping mat of the ill person. It is believed that medicines used in this way can cure or prevent even internal ailments. Clearly, any clinical benefits from remedies so applied that make no contact whatsoever with the ill person, cannot be explained by conventional pharmacological mechanisms. This non-pharmaceutical approach in the appropriate cultural environment and in the acculturated person can have emotion-stabilizing and placebo-enhancing effect, since such a person and his/her caregivers believe in the appropriateness and potency of the treatment. The beneficial effects of such treatment, if any, are not due to magic!

(2) Even when the plant is decocted and administered by the oral route, there is no precise dosage as we know it in modern medicine. The usual instruction is to take a measure of the concoction as required. Such instruction

is more about 'how' the medicine is to be taken, than a description of 'how much' is to be taken.

It is partly for this reason that modern medical scientists claim that TAM practices are imprecise or unorthodox and even dangerous. My inference from TAM theory as described in this book is that while adherence to the rules of dosage is critically important in modern drug therapy, its absence in traditional African medicine usage is also consistent with TAM theory. This pattern of plant use in TAM can be fully justified, both in terms of emotion stabilization being a therapeutic objective, and because poisonous plants were excluded from the pharmacopoeia of traditional remedies.

(3) The criticism by medical scientists that the absence of dosage in TAM invalidates the latter, comes from the medical scientists' experience of using poisonous substances as drugs. There are many important ways in which the use of drugs in modern medicine and the use of plant medicines in TAM, especially when the plant remedy is employed in the treatment of serious illness, differ.

In the first place, in TAM, the plant remedy is supposed to cure the illness. If the expected cure is not apparent in a reasonable period of time, attention shifts to other ideas, for example, consult another healer, use another plant remedy or resort to esoteric measures such as divination and the evocation of the supernatural. In modern medicine on the other hand, the drug prescribed for an illness is quite often meant to control the disease and may have to be taken for life (e.g., anti-diabetic, anti-hypertensive, anti-rheumatic, antiretroviral medicines).

These medicines control the disease but do not cure it. In such cases, accurate dosage is absolutely crucial for success, not only to ensure that the disease is kept under adequate control, but also, just as importantly, to prevent cumulative toxic side effects of the drug during a lifetime of having to take it.

The above argument is not an apology for the failure of traditional healers to prepare their remedies according to modern rules of dosage but a clarification of the reality of the cultural environment from which African medicine evolved. The important point is that the fortuitous exclusion of poisonous plants from the repertoire of African remedies has resulted in medicines that have, in modern terminology, large therapeutic indices (TI) or large safety margins, allowing treatment to proceed without adherence to the strict rules of dosage. The absence of a precise dosage in TAM usage of plant remedies, is an attribute of the system, rather than as a ground for invalidating it as an irrational practice.

But, at the same time, this culture of imprecision has left an imprint on the peoples' subconscious that leads to contradic-tions in their use of modern drugs. These problems arising from what might be called a clash of medical cultures must be recognized and factored into the training of Africa's medical personnel.

Influence of TAM culture on modern medicine practice in Africa: Some observations

Some of the behaviour exhibited by Nigerians when using modern drugs can be explained in terms of attitudes internalized from **TAM** practices. There is a dangerous disregard for the doctor's prescription; though a scarcely documented phenomenon, this is a well known characteristic behaviour among Nigerian patients of all classes. A typical example of this behaviour is illustrated by a true incident recorded by this writer in Delta State.[108]

> On being discharged from the Eku Baptist Hospital, Mr. O.A. (not his real name) was given five different types of drugs (tablets and capsules) in separate little brown envelopes marked with instructions for their use. When I arrived at the hospital to take the old gentleman home, I found to my dismay that he had instructed one of his wives to discharge the contents of the envelopes into one large screw-capped plastic container—to protect the medicines from the rains! How would he take the medicine, now that he had destroyed the doctor's instructions? I asked. He said he would take some from time to time, when he did not feel well. It did not matter which he took, and when, since he would eventually take them all, and in any case, medicine is medicine and they are all going into the same place —his stomach.

To be fair to Mr. O.A., to be prescribed all these medicines after he was well enough to be discharged from hospital, is not what he would expect from his considerable experience

[108] D. T. Okpako, Principles of Pharmacology - A tropical approach (Cambridge, Cambridge University Press, 1991) p. 13.

of herbal treatments in TAM. What were all these medicines for? Each of the five drugs was to be taken by mouth, but each had a different dose schedule, e.g. one capsule was to be taken three times a day, another, two tablets to be taken four times a day, etc.

In TAM, even if one needed to use more than one plant to treat an ailment, the plants would be combined in one concoction, and a measure taken as required until the illness was cured, or until an alternative treatment was sought. Multiple drugs with separate dose schedules in the treatment of an illness is more the rule than the exception in modern medicine, for various reasons which are not always obvious to the traditional African patient; one drug in the prescription may be there to counter the adverse effects, or, to augment the action, of another drug in the prescription. Vitamins or iron tablets for anaemia, may be prescribed for a patient who is being treated with antibiotics for a bacterial infection etc. Doctors, pharma-cists, nurses and others in charge of patient care should not take it for granted that their clients are conversant with these nuances of drug use in modern medicine.

The main reason for the complicated dose schedules in modern medicine is that drugs are poisons, which, if not taken in strictly regulated doses, can be harmful. The idea that the medicine for the treatment of an illness can also be harmful, is an alien thought to someone like Mr. A.O. who would insist that the medicine prescribed by the doctor must be good medicine, which is not supposed to be poisonous. If the expected cure of the illness does not materialize from taking the particular medicine, one can take more, or try another remedy!

The idea that medicine is medicine adversely affects the proper use of modern drugs in another way. For example, the modern doctor's prescription for bacterial or other infections is meant to be complied with for good reasons, an important one being to ensure that the bacteria, viruses or parasites causing the disease are completely eliminated, to avoid the emergence of resistant organisms. But the common experience with many patients is that as soon as they feel relief from the illness they stop taking the medicine. What is more and worse, the patient may dispense the remnants of the drug to family and friends who are ill, sometimes, no matter what they are suffering from.

Thus the attitudes and beliefs internalized from traditional medicine culture underlie the misuse of drugs in modern medicine in Africa. This is one reason why students in African colleges of pharmacy and medicine should be exposed to the basic principles of African medicine as enunciated in this book. It is not enough for the pharmacist to spout "take one tablet, three times a day" and then turn his/her back on the patient. The pharmacist, like the doctor, needs to understand where the patient is coming from, and make the effort to educate him/her on the proper use of modern drugs, so that our huge expenditure on drugs will not go to waste.

In conclusion, we can reiterate that the rules of dosage, as we know them in modern medicine, do not apply in African medicine, is an inherent attribute of the latter, consistent with

    i.   the historical absence of precision technology in the cultures in which the system evolved,

ii. the fact that the pharmacopoeia of traditional
plant remedies excluded overtly poisonous
plants, and

iii. the fact that diffusion of emotional tension
rather than the elimination of a specific cause of
disease, is a core therapeutic objective in
traditional African medicine.

That being the case it is an error to attempt to invalidate
TAM, as biomedical scientists do, on the grounds that the
use of plant remedies in the system do not comply with the
rules of dosage. It is erroneous on the part of biomedical
scientists to attempt a validation of traditional African
medicine by retrospectively invoking principles that have
force in modern medicine.

Chapter 13

The Placebo Effect

I t is useful to devote some space in this book to the phenomenon now known in modern medicine as the placebo effect, which is that any medical intervention including the administration of an inert substance, can lead to the desired improvement in an ill person. This effect, about which much debate has raged in the recent literature of modern medicine, is probably an important component of the clinical response to therapy in TAM, especially in serious life-threatening illnesses. It is important to emphasize here that the placebo effect is an emotional response to therapy, and it is a physiological reality. I am aware that to attribute any part of the clinical benefit of African medicine to a placebo effect is to provoke the charge from certain quarters that one is denying the curative value of African medicine by implying that it is a mere psychological placebo! A significant proportion of the clinical benefit from virtually all therapeutic interventions, including drug therapy in modern medicine, is contributed by the placebo effect.

In TAM, the management of a serious life-threatening illness takes place in an emotionally charged atmosphere. In a situation where the cause, of what appears to be imminent death, cannot be physically ascertained, the people are fearful and anxious. The search for cure is a

SCIENCE INTERROGATING BELIEF

search for spiritual causation, accompanied by elaborate ritual performances (divination, incantations, sacrifices, etc). If, as explained below, the placebo effect is an emotional non-specific response to therapeutic intervention, then we might expect the effect to be highly significant in this system of healing.

In modern medicine, the aim, according to the germ theory of disease, is to identify the physical cause of the illness and to remove it, by poisoning it with a drug or by surgical excision. Consequently, the tendency is to consider the placebo effect as unimportant. In fact the tendency, as we shall see later in this chapter, is to regard the placebo effect as an artifact to be discounted from the total clinical benefit of the intervention, in order to reveal and emphasize the specificity of the treatment offered to the patient. It is important to make this distinction because it is the search for selective toxicity, for an agent that will specifically remove or control the cause of disease that drives drug discovery in the pharmaceutical industry and academic work in university departments of pharmacology and research institutes.

The placebo is an artifact in modern medicine
It is now generally accepted that clinical improvement can result, under suitable conditions, from administering an inert material to a patient. Such clinical improvement that is not due to a specific action of what is given is known as the placebo effect; it is likely to be a wholly emotional relief response to the fact that something positive is being done about an intolerable situation. It is a positive emotional response that should be understood in the context of psychoneuroimmunology which involves a

series of actual physiological mechanisms initiated in the brain, which couple the emotional experience to neural, endocrine and immune defence structures. The placebo effect accompanies the majority of therapeutic interventions. The fact that the detailed physiological mechanism of the placebo effect is not yet known, should not be taken to mean that the effect is an unreal imaginary 'psychological' artifact.

It has been estimated that the placebo effect accounts for between 30 and 60 per cent of the benefit derived from contemporary biomedical procedures.[109] Regulatory authorities know that the placebo effect is a constant component of all drug treatment, that is, the clinical benefit of any drug comes from a combination of the specific action of the drug on its intended target e.g., receptor systems, enzyme or pathogenic microorganism, plus a significant placebo component that is separate from the specific action of the drug. Therefore in clinical trials of new drugs, the placebo effect, which is a nonspecific response to treatment, is regarded as an adulterating artifact, a sort of contaminant that must be subtracted, as it were, in order to reveal the true quality, the specific action, of the new drug. The methods for achieving this objective are phased clinical trials conducted in cooperation with human volunteers. Clinical trials are a series of tests that a new drug must undergo in human subjects following the drug's successful pre-clinical laboratory animal model studies that have established the potential usefulness of the drug for the specified disease.

---

[109] H.K. Beecher, "Surgery as Placebo: a quantitative study of bias". J Am Med Assoc. 1961 (176): 1102-1107; F.M.A. Ukoli, Order Among Parasites, Inaugural lecture, Ibadan University Press, University of Ibadan 1974: 195.

Clinical trials are important to prove that the pre-clinical results can be translated to man in terms of efficacy for the specified disease and to demonstrate that the drug is safe for use in humans in the specified dose range.

Clinical trials are legal requirements set up by drug regulatory authorities that a new drug must successfully undergo before its approval for general use. The trial design is technically called randomized double-blind placebo-controlled clinical trial (randomized controlled trials [RCT] for short) in which the drug is tested for efficacy and safety on groups of adult-consenting participants arranged in such a way as to minimize bias. A characteristic feature of the design is that neither the patients recruited into the trial nor the people (nurses and doctors) administering the trial know which, e.g. tablets, capsules, injections etc, contain the 'active' drug and which are a dummy preparation disguised as the drug, also known as the placebo. One person, the director of the trial programme who will remove the blindfold from the data for statistical analysis, knows!

Clinical improvement in the patients taking the 'active' drug must be significantly greater than the improvement in those taking the placebo, otherwise the new drug will not merit registration as a therapeutic agent for the specified disease. The point to emphasize is that in these clinical trials, the dummy tablet, that is, the placebo, is found to always produce a clinical relief or cure. What the regulatory authorities insist on is that the 'active' drug's clinical benefit must be significantly greater than that of the dummy if the new drug is to merit registration. The significantly greater clinical benefit of an acceptable drug is attributed to the selective toxicity, the specific action, of its active principles at the identified cause of disease.

It may help to clarify the point by citing a general example of how the system works. In the early 1970s, James Black and his team of researchers at Smyth-Kline & French laboratories in London discovered the drug cimetidine, a selective antagonist at histamine H_2-receptors which they hoped would be useful in the treatment of stomach ulcer. H_2-receptors are the receptors on which histamine acts to increase gastric acid secretion thereby causing stomach ulcer disease. Before regulatory authorities could register approval for cimetidine for the treatment of gastric ulcer, it had to be shown in RCTs that the clinical effect of the drug in ulcer patients was significantly better than that of a dummy tablet, the placebo, statistically. The superiority of cimetidine in the trial and hence its acceptance as a good anti-ulcer drug is predicated on the body of scientific evidence that it specifically blocks (inactivates, poisons) histamine H_2-receptors. The point that I am making is that some of the patients who received the placebo tablets in this trial, the tablets that did not contain an active H_2-receptor blocking drug also experienced clinical relief from their ulcer disease; but cimetidine was statistically superior to the placebo in these trials. Hence cimetidine (brand name, Tagamet) was registered as a new anti-ulcer drug.

The placebo effect is an emotional response attributed to the belief that the remedy will be effective in the condition being treated. In a frequently quoted study[110]

---

[110] H. Benson, M.D. Epstein, The placebo effect: A neglected asset in the care of patients. JAMA, 1975, (232): 1225-1227.

the authors found that there was a consistent pattern of 70-80% effectiveness reported initially by enthusiasts of a particular form of therapy, e.g., a new drug, psychoanalytic intervention or alternative therapy. When sceptics or non-enthusiasts (non believers) were recruited into the same trial scheme, the reported effectiveness dropped to 30-60%. The difference was the belief factor in the placebo effect. The placebo effect is greatest when both doctor and patient believe in the efficacy of the proposed treatment.[111] The authority of the prescriber—white coat/stethoscope (the ritual attire of the doctor) increases the placebo effect, as does the personality of the patient. Attributes of the 'placebo personality' have been described as over-anxiety, emotional dependence and immaturity.[112] In situations of life-threatening illness, most human beings display all or some of these attributes.

Even in surgery where clinical improvement is presumed to be due to mechanical repair, Moerman[113] concluded from a review of several cases that 'although coronary bypass surgery works, it does not necessarily work for the reasons that it is done'. Several coronary bypass patients experienced dramatic symptomatic improvements after the surgery, even when the new bypass did not function. In concluding that the placebo effect

---

[111] H. Benson & D.P. McCallie Jr. Angina pectoris and the placebo effect. New England Journal of Medicine 1979 (300): 1424-1429.

[112] H.M. Adler and V.B.O. Hammett, The doctor-patient relationship revisited: an analysis of the placebo effect. Annals of Internal Medicine. 1973; (78): 595-598.

[113] D.E. Moerman, Physiology and symbols: the anthropological implications of the placebo effect, in: L. Romanucci-Ross, D.E. Moerman and L.R. Tancredi, editors, The Anthropology of Medicine (New York: Praeger, 1983).

must be partly responsible for the observed symptomatic improvement, Moerman points out that neurological impulses and emotional stress contribute to the coronary artery spasm, and that "angina and heart attack are the results of mental processes...subject to symbolic influences."

What does RCT achieve?

A positive RCT establishes for a drug, that more of its clinical benefit comes from a specific pharmacological mechanism than from a general nonspecific placebo effect. But RCT does not remove the placebo effect, this being a constant component of the clinical benefit of any drug. The new drug is then promoted in conferences and the media for doctors, pharmacists, nurses and enlightened patients to know that a new drug with high specific action for the particular disease has just been approved. This is backed by the scientific evidence. The facts of the scientifically proven specificity of the drug for the disease condition, its approval for general use by the powerful regulatory authorities, e.g., the Food and Drug Administration (FDA) of America, and its promotion by the industry to that effect must increase the belief of doctors in general practice, specialist doctors and patients alike in the efficacy of the new drug, thereby, increasing the placebo effect of the drug when it is in general use. Thus, not only do double blind clinical trials not remove the placebo effect of the drug, the trials, if successful, must actually directly contribute to enhancing the placebo effect because the trial increases the range of believers in its efficacy.

The question has been asked, of modern medicine, that if the placebo effect is clinically beneficial, and it is a constant in the clinical benefit of therapy, then why has the effect not been harnessed directly for human benefit[114] instead of regarding it, as we do now, as an unwanted artifact? After all, a placebo-derived clinical effect would be the ideal therapy. It would have no side effects! If the placebo effect could be maximized, it would be the safest of all treatments of disease. Yet there is no evidence that any attempt has been made in modern medicine to harness the placebo effect for human benefit.

But with the entrenched pharmacological theory of selective toxicity as the paradigm for how a drug should work, and the powerful pharmaceutical industries that depend on that theory for drug discovery and profits, it is unlikely that the placebo effect will be harnessed for therapeutic purposes any time soon.

The placebo effect is not an artifact in traditional African medicine

Traditional African medicine seems to be a method of healing in which the placebo effect is not looked upon as an artifact; if anything it is actively mobilized when treating serious illnesses. Hence, the placebo is probably of greater quantitative significance in TAM than it is in modern medicine. By that I mean that the contribution of the nonspecific placebo effect to any clinical benefit achieved by all treatment procedures in African medicine is likely to be greater than it is in modern medicine, where

---

[114] J.M. Pearce, The placebo enigma. Quarterly Journal of Medicine 1995 (88): 215- 220.

the selective poisoning of the cause of disease by the drug is the desired goal.

In African medicine emotional distress is believed to underpin serious illness and, the placebo effect is, as far as can be ascertained, at least partly an emotional response and therefore likely to be a contributing factor in clinical relief from illness in this system. Traditional African medicine enthusiasts usually disagree strongly with this view, preferring to think that African plant remedies must contain drug-like entities with disease-specific therapeutic properties. To suggest that the placebo effect may contribute to their usefulness is to imply that these treatments are mere worthless placebos, and thereby somehow diminish the African medical heritage. The fact that we have not been able to establish scientific proof of their specificity does not mean that traditional treatments are mere placebos, they further argue.

My counter argument, is that the beneficial clinical response to nonspecific treatment, called the placebo effect, is real and important; it is only in modern medicine that this response is looked down upon as a mere worthless artifact. Traditional healing systems recognized what modern medicine now calls "the placebo effect" as an important element in therapeutic interventions, and took steps to maximize it; and there is no evidence that in general use, the placebo effect is not a significant component of the clinical benefit which the patient derives from modern drugs.

The "mere placebo" attitude comes from exposure to the principles of modern medicine where the drug must have a specific activity against a causative agent to be of value. The principle of specificity of drug action in modern medicine is so powerful that it overwhelms the indisputable fact that the placebo nonspecific effect is a constant and significant proportion of any drug's total clinical benefit. In other words, however important the selective action of a drug may be as a mechanism for controlling/curing a disease, when that drug is used as therapy, the placebo always contributes its own quota for the clinical benefit of the drug. As has been pointed out earlier, this quota is estimated to be 30-60% of the therapeutic benefit of medication. This effect may in fact be the only certain clinical effect that may be left of a drug after heat-, and humidity-, driven deteriorations of active ingredients left in containers in sea or airports in the tropics; or of drugs sold in open markets and bus stations in Nigeria, not to talk of fake drugs without active ingredients.[115] The placebo effect is always there as a constant. This has been demonstrated over and over again in clinical trials in modern medicine. It may not be enough to save a patient from serious illness, but it is there, and any process that enhances its contribution therapy should be seriously appraised.

As shown in earlier chapters, serious illness in TAM has its roots in sustained emotional distress, and all therapeutic procedures including the use of plant remedies, are accompanied by emotionally charged rituals such as incantations, divination, confessions and ritual sacrifices, etc. My point is that the effect of these procedures is to douse emotional tension in the sick person, and to enhance confidence and belief in the

---

[115] D.T. Okpako, Principles of Pharmacology—A tropical approach (Cambridge, Cambridge University Press, 1991) p. 41.

efficacy of the treatment being offered. In the emotionally charged atmosphere of a life-threatening illness in African medicine, a general acceptance that the ritual procedures adopted towards healing are culturally appropriate and the belief that the remedy will be efficacious are all factors that maximize the placebo effect of therapy.

Clinical trials like incantations, contribute to the placebo effect

Incantations and other rituals deployed in TAM consolidate the acculturated African's belief in the efficacy of the treatment being given. As indicated already, clinical trials in modern medicine do the same, in this case by demonstrating that the clinical benefit of the drug comes from its selective action on the cause of disease. In modern medicine establishing the quantitative supremacy of specific action over the placebo effect of a medication, is the desired objective in drug development. For the purpose of this argument, we can say that the elaborate clinical trial exercise is a 'ritual performance'; once it has been executed to the satisfaction of the acculturated participants (medical profession), the belief in the efficacy of the drug is consolidated. The clinical trial is a form of incantation.

The belief among participants in TAM is that incantation brings out the healing power of the remedy; it is therefore an appropriate accompaniment to medication. Incantation must add to the placebo effect of treatment, so that even when the medication is most unlikely to have a significant specific effect on the cause of the disease (as for example, when the medication is applied to the patient's surroundings, without direct contact with the individual), the medication is believed to be able to cure an illness due to an internal disease.

It can be argued that incantation in African medicine and the double blind placebo controlled clinical trial in modern medicine both enhance the placebo effect of medication by the respective mechanisms enunciated above. In modern medicine we play down the significance of the placebo effect in order to emphasize that the drug's selective toxicity is its mode of action. This ensures the general acceptability of the drug among doctors and regulatory authorities. In TAM we maximize the placebo effect through incantations and other rituals, to the same effect, namely, the general acceptability of the treatment in the acculturated population.

The placebo effect has to be the explanation for any clinical benefits due to remedies that are administered by non-pharmaceutical routes, e.g., remedies encapsulated in a cloth or leather pouch and worn as necklaces, amulets in a waistband or placed under the patient's pillow or lintel of the door to the ill person's room. My strong hunch is that the placebo effect is of greater quantitative significance in African medicine than it is in modern medicine. But the bottom line is the placebo effect contributes to the beneficial clinical relief in both modern and traditional African medicine.

Mechanism of action of plant remedies in African medicine

It may be concluded that plant medicines used in the management of serious illness in African medicine may act in the following ways to produce clinical benefits:

i.   The placebo effect energized by procedures such as incantation, divination, confession and sacrifice that enhance the faith in the treatment scheme

ii. Synergism of effects: Many plants contain a variety of immune-modulators, antioxidants, nutritive elements, anti-inflammatory agents e.g. flavonoids, therapeutic aromas, etc, that may contribute to healing.

iii. Appropriate pharmacological constituents: Despite my contention that the clinical benefit from a plant medicine used in the treatment of chronic life-threatening illness of unknown cause in TAM need not correlate with its pharmacology (i.e., the plant need not contain chemical entities that are selectively toxic to the cause of disease), that the placebo effect may be a significant part of the clinical benefit of plant remedies as they are used in African medicine. I am aware of several instances where important drugs with appropriate pharmacology have been serendipitously discovered in traditional medicine, such as quinine, aspirin and reserpine

This possibility should always be borne in mind in medicinal plant research so that every plant extract is screened for as wide a range of pharmacological activities as possible.

The placebo effect in homeopathy

In homeopathic theory, the potency of the medicine is said to increase with dilution. This is antithetic to pharmacological theory, according to which a drug effect increases with its concentration. A.J. Clark, a pharmacologist with a mathematical tendency, who is often referred to as the father of quantitative pharmacology, has been said to have described homeopathic theory as absurd and demonstrated this by showing that a remedy diluted to the 30th of its potency would contain about one molecule of the active drug in a sphere with a circumference equal to the orbit of Venus! In other words, at very high dilutions, when the drug is supposed to be most potent according to homeopathic theory, the active ingredient is not present!

Controversy between conventional medical scientists and homeopaths has raged for decades. The former argue that at very high or ultra-molecular dilutions (high potencies in homeopathic prescriptions) the drug has been diluted out. Therefore the only explanation for its clinical benefit at this level of dilution must be the placebo effect. In a recent heated exchange, Edzard Ernst[116] described a homeopathic medication as, at best a "helpful placebo" or worse "an unethical intervention".

Homeopaths disagree, claiming that dilution releases the energy in the drug molecule. The higher the dilution the greater the amount of energy released into the diluents and that the homeopathic medicine "might interact with the body energetically rather than chemically".[117] A great deal is known about chemical interactions between elements in the human body and drugs, but little is known about so-called "energetic" interactions.

---

[116] E. Ernst, No to placebo effect. The Guardian 22 February 2010; E. Ernst, Homeopathy, a helpful placebo or an unethical intervention? Trends in Pharmacol. Sci. 2010 (31).

[117] P. Ross, Homeopathy, a helpful placebo or an unethical intervention? Edzard Ernst reply, Trends in Pharmacol. Sci. 2010 (31): 297.

The description of homeopathic practice as an 'unethical intervention' by Ernst above requires comment here. My contention in this book is that in traditional African medicine, much sympathetic attention is paid to the ill person (in fact the patient is the centre of attention, not the disease). This and ritual performances are important elements in the management of serious illness (chronic life-threatening illness of unknown cause). Therefore the placebo effect may be a critically important factor in this healing system.

Do ethical questions arise in traditional African medicine practices, when traditional healers use ritual methods to enhance belief in their treatment procedures? As in all human endeavours the likelihood that some individual practitioners might take advantage of the anxiety and fear of death prevailing in conditions of serious illness, and the gullibility of participants, to cut corners dishonestly cannot be ruled out, but I shall suggest below that deceit was not the purpose in the use of esoteric methods in the resolution of serious illness in African medicine.

The unethical intervention argument by Professor Ernst above rests on two legs:

i. It is unethical, deceitful, to convey to a patient the impression that the medicine that has been given, is specific for the disease when there is, in fact, no proof in the case of homeopathic prescriptions that this is so.

ii. Homeopathic treatment may prevent the patient or relatives from seeking access to good, available and specific drugs that can save the patient's life. There are well publicized cases where such denial of access has happened with disastrous consequences to the patient.

In the TAM treatment of serious illness, the use of elaborate rituals performed to the full knowledge of the patient and caregivers in a cultural environment in which everyone accepts these rituals to be necessary and appropriate, would enhance the placebo mechanism, bearing in mind the belief that serious illness has its origins in sustained emotional distress. In these circumstances, the question whether the treatment is unethical or deceitful does not arise.

The traditional healer would be acting unethically and deceitfully, if he knew that there was a specifically acting alternative remedy or treatment to the one he was giving the patient, while denying him that alternative for an ulterior motive. That is not the case in TAM. The deployment of culturally appropriate procedures which I suggest must enhance the confidence and belief in the treatment being given is simply an attribute of the system. Satisfying cultural norms is how serious illness ought to be dealt with. It so happens that, in modern medicine terminology, this strategy would maximize what is known as the placebo effect of treatment.

From these considerations I propose the following general principle:

> Placebo and selective toxicity are two extremes in a spectrum in the mode of action of medicines in bringing clinical benefit to an ill person; between the two extremes, medicines can have different proportions of each mode depending on the cultural environment and type and method of administration of the

medicine. Plant remedies used in the treatment
of life-threatening illness in TAM may veer
more to the placebo side of the spectrum than
drugs used in modern medicine.

It is worth repeating that the placebo effect is not an
imagined clinical response, but a real physiological
response to emotion, mediated most probably by a
coordinated action of the nervous, endocrine and
immune systems.

The fact that the placebo effect is a constant
component of the response to drug therapy is attested to
in double blind placebo controlled clinical trials
worldwide, where the placebo dummy preparation always
produces a measurable clinical improvement. The fact
that we do not yet have a definitive mechanistic
explanation of this phenomenon does not diminish its
reality.

Traditional African medicine seems to be one healing
method in which the placebo effect is actively co-opted
through elaborate rituals consistent with the theory that
serious illness has its origins in the mind, whereas
modern medicine plays down the placebo effect because
the aim in the latter is to control disease by selectively
attenuating its cause. In both systems, practice is
consistent with theory.

My aim here, as elsewhere in the book, has been to
demonstrate that reason, borne out of intuition,
observation and experience guided the emergence of the
beliefs and practices in African medicine. In the absence
of precision technology, African ancients came to
understand that, what is now called the placebo effect was

an important component of therapy, and that this could be enhanced by ritual perfor-mances, which incidentally served other functions. The fact that the ancients came to that conclusion and incorporated the idea into their healing practices ought to be recognized as a seminal achievement in the history of medical thought.

Chapter 14

Does Traditional Medicine Have a Future in Africa?

A t this stage, let me very briefly summarize what we have learnt from Parts 1 and 2 as a prelude to an answer to the title of this chapter. Ancestor spirit anger and other beliefs in TAM are concepts that underpin the African knowledge of life in small-scale, closely-knit communities. In such communities the people learnt from experience that certain types of immorality represented a threat to their harmonious survival as a cohesive society in which members generally acted in one another's best interests. It was to prevent such potentially destructive antisocial conduct by its members that the ancestor spirit anger belief evolved. In this belief, a life-threatening illness was thought to be inflicted on a member by the ancestors for immoral conduct/antisocial behaviour. In the acculturated individual who shares these inherent beliefs, the commission of such a "sin" could provoke an emotional upheaval in the sinner which in turn could render him/her more prone to serious illness than someone not burdened by such emotions. The main thrust of this book is that this interpretation of ancestor spirit anger should enable us to bring important aspects of TAM under scientific scrutiny and to ways in which modern medicine can benefit from the ideas embedded in the beliefs and methods of the ancient art.

TAM is a healing system that evolved for the benefit of humanity in Africa and which may well contain the primordial origins of ideas concerning the fundamental nature of human illness. But, the question is what to do with these ideas in present day Africa. In other words, what is the future of traditional medicine in Africa?

Conflicting ideas about the way forward

Traditional medicine is practised widely in Africa, but the absence of an articulated theory has made it difficult to put this mode of healing on a systematic professional footing. Indeed traditional African medicine has been so pounded by external influences that, it is said to have lost much of its original focus and is no longer recognizable as a distinct "system" of healing.[118]

In the absence of a written philosophy, its original guiding principles lie vaguely hidden in the distant past. Therefore, despite efforts by governments to promote TAM in order to increase its wider usefulness, nothing more tangible than attempts to professionalize it has resulted. Associations and bureaucracies of traditional medicine have sprung up in urban centres. These are dominated by urban 'educated elite herbalists' most of whom have very little acquaintance with the traditional beliefs or principles that originally formed the basis of traditional herbal practice. As Staugart pointed out, this is a dangerous trend, an "incitement for traditional healers

---

[118] Murray Last, The professionalization of African medicine: Ambiguities and definitions. in: The Professionalisation of African Medicine. M. Last and G. L. Chavunduka, editors (Manchester, Manchester University Press, 1986) p. 1-26.

to adopt successively, the ideas and practices of the biomedical profes-sion, thereby defecting from their own holistic traditions". [119]

Two conflicting ideas have emerged from TAM scholars and enthusiasts:

(a) that traditional healers should be trained in basic sciences to improve their performance, and

(b) that the principles of traditional African medicine should be included in the curricula for the training of doctors, pharmacists, nurses and other health related professionals.

These ideas are symbolic of the struggle for relevance of the two ideologically (or should I say paradigmatically?) opposed systems of health care that exist in Africa, namely, traditional and modern medicine. Those, like this writer, who are sceptical of the view that traditional healers be taught some rudiments of modern medical technology, so that they can, e.g., measure out their remedies in precise quantities in an attempt to adhere to the rules of dosage as in modern medicine, argue that if we did that, we would simply create another cadre of paramedic who must come under the control of the modern doctor, thereby burying the methods and theories of traditional African medicine, and denying ourselves and the rest of the world the potential contributions which lie in these methods. For example, we have learnt from this study so far, that serious illness in one member in a traditional African community was seen as a fundamental threat to the moral and social cohesion of the whole

[119] F. Stautgart, Traditional health care in Botswana, in: Professionalization of African Medicine.   M. Last and G. L. Chavunduka, editors, (Manchester, Manchester University Press, 1986).

community. This meant that there was a wider community involvement in the search for a solution than is the case in modern medicine, where illness is the isolated concern of the sufferer and the immediate family. This is a fundamental idea that those who formulate health policies for Africa should take on board; health care should be a matter in which every one in society should be an active participant in terms of policy formulation and implementation, not a top down affair for the privileged who can afford to benefit from it.

On the other hand, including TAM principles in the curricula of our colleges of medicine and pharmacy, is an idea that I would strongly espouse. For one thing, the modern Nigerian health care provider deals with clients whose attitudes to illness are rooted in traditional beliefs of the type discussed in this book. Many of the people who eventually come to see the modern doctor hold these beliefs, whether they openly admit it or not. It would seem logical that the modern medical practitioner should be intellectually equipped to at least understand the alternative views brought into the illness situation, for the benefit of the patient. For another thing, the idea that emotional factors play a key role in the occurrence of illness and in healing, which is profoundly enunciated in TAM, should be a prominent aspect of modern medicine practice in Africa. The study of critical elements of psychoneuro-immunology or brain control of host defence should be given emphasis in the curricula of colleges of medicine and pharmacy in Africa, if not at undergraduate, then certainly at an appropriate postgraduate specialty level.

Can African medicine be professionalized?

An important issue is what to do about traditional healers and the traditional healing profession in Africa. At the moment every traditional healer is law unto himself/herself, practising the art and improvising more or less as he has done in his own lineage for generations. One suggestion is that steps should be taken to systematize the traditional healers' practice; to ground it on generally accepted principles. It is on the basis of such principles, it is argued, that ethical guidelines can be prescribed and new entrants recruited into its practice. Without that, it is further argued, TAM cannot develop the attributes of a coherent profession, and in time TAM would dissipate into extinction.

The question is, can traditional healers come together to formulate a basis for such systematization to achieve professional status, without succumbing to the temptation to unduly commercialize the practice? What I have proposed in this book represents a theoretical framework around which a systematic curriculum and professional structure for TAM can be built.

The future of traditional medicine in Africa

Given the tremendous advances being made on all fronts in the medical sciences; and given that modern medical facilities will, even if slowly, become more and more widely available throughout Africa, it is unlikely that traditional African medicine and its authentic practitioners will survive in their present form into the next century. Traditional African medicine thus falls into the category of traditional African cultural institutions and practices (e.g. religious institutions and related practices) whose further development was abrogated by European presence. Negative representations of these institutions and practices in European colonial literature, and their uncritical substitution with 'modern' practices led to their demise. This prevented autochthonous changes to these cultural practices that might have modified aspects of the practice or that might have led to the abandonment of it in the light of prevailing experience, from taking place in a time frame that would have allowed society to adjust accordingly. So we will never know how traditional African medicine would have evolved had 'natural selection' been allowed to prevail. The demise of traditional African institutions under the pressure of European propaganda had nothing to do with the Darwinian survival of the fittest principle, as some would claim. Traditional institutions did not have a fair chance of survival.

Now, among educated Africans—the leaders of thought— one can discern different tendencies towards traditional African cultural practices. One tendency is a nationalistic acceptance and defence of these practices as African heritage without critical appraisal, in reaction to the years of their denigration in colonialist writings. Another is total rejection of the African past as worthless in a rush to catch up with the West, plus a variety of mixtures of attitudes in between.

The view of this writer is that traditional cultural practices evolved from the accumulated experience and understanding of human behaviour in, and knowledge of, the African environment. The practices were thus underpinned by rational thought, expressed in appropriate symbols and metaphors. The cultural practices did not arise from superstitious irrational instincts as the colonial literature tended to portray them. A common cliché is 'culture is dynamic'; as the African environment has changed over time, and the people have become more and more exposed to other peoples' ideas and influences, traditional cultural practices must change. This has happened to cultures throughout human history. What we must ensure is that we, to borrow another cliché, 'do not throw out the baby with the bath water'.

The task before the educated African therefore is to use all available tools to seriously examine the past and bring out what is best in it into the open to invigorate the present, to add the African perspective to the human development project. What we can learn from the past, ironically, is embedded in the beliefs and practices that were traditionally described in the colonial press as "mumbo- jumbo" superstition; but it is through the examination of these beliefs that we can learn from the African past. I hope that this book can be an example of such an inquiry in the area of health care.

PART THREE

Treatment of Minor Ailments in Traditional African Medicine

Most Africans in malaria endemic areas were partially immune to the disease; to them the disease was a minor ailment presenting as fever, aches and pains which they treated with herbal medicines. In the partially immune person such treatment amounted to clinical cure of the disease. This hypothesis is discussed extensively in this part of the book, in the light of current knowledge of malaria pathology and eradication strategies in Africa.

Chapter 15

Treatment of Minor Ailments in Traditional African Medicine: Malaria as a case study

B iomedical scientists often describe TAM practices as mystical, magical, irrational and superstitious. This is almost certainly because the esoteric beliefs and concepts that are evoked as explanations for the occurrence of serious illness and, for its prevention and treatment have no apparent scientific rational equivalents in modern medicine. So far in this book we have tried to show that such beliefs and methods are rational and consistent with the assumptions that indigenous Africans make about the causes of life-threatening illnesses.

But such beliefs and methods are not called upon when indigenous Africans treat minor ailments with plant remedies and, this aspect of African medicine requiring no esoteric consultations, no divination, no incantation, is what the people practice most of the time. Modern medicine has something to learn also from the traditional Africans' use of herbal remedies. For example, traditional herbal medicine is practised against the background of TAM's basic principles, which are essentially different from those of modern medicine and explains why there are methodological differences in the use of African herbal remedies and in the use of drugs in modern medicine. Therefore it is erroneous to evaluate the use of plant remedies in TAM on the basis of principles that have force in modern medicine, as modern medical practitioners tend to. A case in point is the usual assertion by the latter that the validity of African medicine is questionable because the practitioners do not adhere to strict rules of dosage when using herbal remedies. In this regard, it can be argued that the use of herbal remedies in TAM should be evaluated only in the context of the core principles of the system. This argument also applies to the use of herbal remedies in the treatment of minor ailments.

In TAM, the use of plant remedies to treat minor ailments is an entirely common-sense practice, similar to the use of non-prescription OTC drugs such as paracetamol to treat self-diagnosed minor ailments in modern medicine. What is intriguing and remarkable is how prescience societies came to know appropriate plant remedies for the treatment of the common ailments that troubled them most frequently.

Malaria was a minor ailment in Africa

Malaria, now a high profile disease in Africa, is an example of a disease which indigenous Africans successfully treated as a minor ailment in before the colonial period. ~~ancient times.~~ Common symptoms of malaria are fever, aches and pains. Even though the people did not recognize the parasitic origin of malaria, they were familiar with its symptoms which they treated with commonly available herbal remedies that were in all probability, efficacious. As matters have turned out, new research in biomedicine and malaria have revealed findings, which on the whole, validate the peoples' traditional treatment of malaria. The scientific evidence is:

i. the herbal remedies commonly used by indigenous people to treat fever, aches and pains, possess anti-inflammatory properties, and

ii. inflammation mechanisms contribute significantly to malaria. This convergence of traditional African intuition and scientific evidence is expatiated upon in the rest of the book. The fact that prescience indigenous African societies could have arrived at the knowledge and use of plants possessing anti-inflammatory properties for the treatment of malaria is a remarkable indication of how Mother Nature reveals herself to those close to her; and it is one reason why throughout this book, that this writer has insisted that we have a duty to humanity to scrutinize African traditional knowledge systems for meaning and relevance in the light of prevailing scientific experience. It is also surprising that current modern medicine approaches to malaria eradication do not refer to this knowledge and the accumulated experience of coping with malaria in indigenous African populations.

Why malaria could be treated as a minor ailment among indigenous African populations

Malaria disease was a minor ailment among indigenous African populations, and therefore amenable to successful treatment with anti-fever remedies. Two supporting explanations are as follows:

  i. the peoples' partial immunity to the disease (partial immunity is defined below) and

  ii. the peoples' herbal remedies possessed anti-inflammatory properties.

Partial immunity. Traditional African herbal treatment of malaria was successful in the partially immune African almost certainly because the immune system of the infected person was primed to clear the parasite once the inflammation was effectively treated. Of the wide variety of pathogenic microorganisms to which Africans in their hygienically basic environments were exposed, none can be said to have this attribute of inducing immunity to a greater degree than the Plasmodium falciparum parasite. This was because without it, as we know now, the infection caused by this parasite was fatal; Africans living in endemic areas were therefore specially adapted to it in evolutionary time.

Herbal remedies, however, would not be a successful malaria treatment in the non-immune or immunologically compromised person, including Europeans making first-time contact with the disease, persons living with HIV/AIDS, and even indigenous Africans returning home after years of sojourn in malaria-free countries of Europe and America or Africans now living in houses with mosquito-netted windows or sleeping under insecticide-impregnated nets and are thus protected from frequent contact with the malaria parasite. In such persons, traditional herbal remedies would not be an adequate treatment for malaria.

What I shall keep emphasizing therefore is that partial immunity is what we are compelled to evoke as underscoring the historical success of such treatments in the Africans living in malaria endemic areas. One observation which kept recurring in the accounts of early Europeans to West Africa, many of whom died from malaria, was that Africans were immune to malaria. They were not totally immune, but partial immunity was enough to prevent them from dying in the same numbers as the Europeans. [120]

Why did the WHO not factor partial immunity and traditional African herbal treatment into malaria control strategies?

The World Health Organization (WHO) is the world's expert on health issues. Its subcommittee, the Tropical Diseases Research Programme (TDR) is the think tank on research funding for malaria and a selected group of tropical diseases worldwide. In the past four decades these institutions have devoted more brains and funds to malaria research than at any previous period in the history of the war against malaria. It would thus surprise anyone who cares to reflect on this problem to find that throughout this effort, these bodies seem not to have sought answers to such basic questions as, how did Africans who have lived with this disease from the beginning of time manage to survive? And, if indeed the question was asked, why were its findings not factored into its malaria control and treatment strategies? From

---

[120] David Okpako, Malaria and Indigenous Knowledge in Africa, (Ibadan University Press, Ibadan, 2011).

254   SCIENCE INTERROGATING BELIEF

what follows in this section of the book, it is apparent that
if the WHO had incorporated the African experience of
malaria in its plans and recommendations, the outcome
would be different from what we see today. A disease that
was apparently successfully treated as a minor ailment in
indigenous African populations has become a dangerous
disease, now described as an epidemic in apocalyptic
terms. That malaria has become a major health problem
among indigenous African populations can be attributed
to   modern   chemotherapeutic   interventions   with
plasmodicidal anti-malaria drugs.

   One can speculate as to why the WHO and the
experts that dominate its scientific thinking on malaria
would not have considered the indigenous African
treatment of the disease as priority as follows: From the
15th century onwards, malaria killed hundreds of
Europeans who came in contact with the disease for the
first time. This earned West Africa the terrifying epitaph
of "the white man's grave".[121] The fear of malaria as a
deadly disease and the idea that Africans were immune to
it, has dominated European thinking since colonial times.
The advice from colonial scientists at the London and
Liverpool Schools of Hygiene and Tropical Medicine
and their counterparts in France, Berlin and other
colonizing metropolises, was that the best strategy for
Europeans to prevent death from malaria was to treat the
disease with quinine—the first anti-malaria drug with
plasmodicidal action (it kills the plasmodium parasite),
reduce contact with the anopheles mosquito by sleeping

[121] Adelola Adeloye, African Pioneers of Modern Medicine. Nigerian doctors of the
nineteenth century, (Ibadan: University Press Ltd, 1985).

under mosquito nets and maintain a good distance from the 'natives' who were presumed to be immune to the disease but were carriers of the deadly parasite (hence boys quarters were invented).

The current strategies under the WHO-inspired Roll Back Malaria Programme[122] are not fundamentally different from the colonial scientists' advice of the early 19th century. This suggests that the old European fear of malaria remains a critical factor in the options preferred by WHO when considering malaria control strategies. Added to this is an overlay of the difficult-to-eradicate notion, propagated in colonial literature and internalized by educated Africans, that traditional African institutions and knowledge systems have little or no value or relevance to today's problems.

Malaria is an ancient malady with which Africans in endemic areas lived in biological equilibrium from the beginning of time. There is no evidence that malaria was about to extinguish the African population before modern chemotherapy came to the rescue! If anything, it is modern chemotherapy and the resulting multi-drug resistant malaria parasite that has, during the past three or four decades, increased the virulence of Plasmodium falciparum and changed the disease from a minor ailment to a major deadly disease, a problem that now requires complete rethinking.

What has been proposed above is that the partial immunity of indigenous African people to malaria accounted for the probable success of herbal remedies in the traditional treatment of the disease. It would

---

[122] Okpako, 2011, 120.

therefore be helpful to briefly describe the different elements that constitute what I have referred to as partial immunity.

Partial immunity of the African to malaria

By partial immunity in the resident West African I am referring to the many adaptive mechanisms, which can be said to have been induced by the most deadly of the malaria parasites, Plasmodium falciparum, to protect its host from the disease caused by its presence, which also ensured that the parasite did not self-destruct.[123] These mechanisms include acquired immunity and the many well-studied genetic adaptations that enabled the African people to live in biological equilibrium with malaria. The following is a very brief description of important examples of those protective adaptations.

i.   Acquired immunity to malaria

There is evidence that adult West Africans, as a result of frequent contact with Plasmodium falciparum, have acquired a certain level of resistance to malaria disease. Research done in the 1950s at the University of Ibadan, showed that compared to Europeans, West Africans have very high plasma concentra-tions of gamma globulins compared to Caucasians.[124] Gamma globulins are a group of plasma proteins which include antibodies to malaria parasite antigens in a person repeatedly exposed to

---

[123] Ukoli, 1974.

[124] J.C. Edozien, The serum proteins of healthy adult Nigerians. J Clin Pathol. 1957 Aug;10 (3): 276-279.

anopheles mosquito bites. People of West African origin living in the Diaspora also have this characteristic hypergammaglobinaemia compared to their host Caucasians, but it is West Africans normally resident in malaria endemic areas that have the highest concentration of this protein. After prolonged residence of West Africans in a malaria-free environment (e.g., London) the plasma concentration of this protein falls, but it returns to its normal high levels when such individuals return to West Africa with renewed contact with the falciparum parasite, suggesting that hypergammaglobinaemia and the capacity to raise the concentration of the protein when the need arises, is a genetically-driven protective mechanism in people living in close proximity, and repeatedly exposed, to parasitic infection. In other words West Africans are genetically primed to raise their gammaglobulin concentrations (antibodies to plasmodium antigens) on contact with malaria parasite infections.

What this suggests is that the resident West African is in an active state of readiness to immunologically respond to the presence of the malaria parasite. In such a person, the successful herbal treatment of malaria-induced fever is enough to cure the disease. Herbal treatment as such would not eliminate the parasite, but the ensuing surge in immune activity following such treatment would eliminate the parasite or reduce parasitaemia to a harmless level, in the person with partial immunity. This hypothesis has not been directly validated, other than the fact that many people in both rural and urban centres in Nigeria do treat themselves when they have fever, aches and pains with herbal remedies. The proposition is plausible and it can be tested.

ii. Glucose-6-phosphate dehydrogenase deficiency

Glucose-6-phosphate dehydrogenase (G6PD) is an enzyme whose important function is to maintain the integrity of the red blood cell membrane by protecting it from the damaging effects of oxidative stress caused by reactive oxygen radicals produced in the body during normal metabolism. About a quarter of Nigerians have genetic G6PD deficiency, that is, they are born without the enzyme. G6PD deficiency itself is not a disease, but people who are deficient may be susceptible to severe haemolysis if they eat certain foods (e.g. fava beans) or take certain types of drug such as the sulphonamides.

A G6PD deficiency is thought to partially protect the deficient person from Plasmodium falciparum malaria,[125] but not from malaria disease caused by other plasmodia. The hypothesis is supported by three kinds of evidence: First, G6PD deficiency is found among people who live or whose ancestors lived in regions of the world where P. falciparum malaria is, or has been, endemic. Thus G6PD deficiency is of high frequency in sub-Saharan Africa and it occurs in Arabia and Iran, the Mediterranean basin (Turkey, Greece, Italy, Sicily), the Indian subcontinent and South East Asia. The trans-Atlantic slave trade and migration have caused the G6PD deficient gene to spread to the Caribbean, the Americas and the British Isles. This so-called "geographical coincidence" is the

---

[125] L. Luzzatto, Genetics of red cells and susceptibility to malaria. Blood, 1979 (54): 961–976.

backbone of the hypothesis that the gene deficiency was an evolutionary protective adaptation against the deadly P. falciparum malaria. Geographical coincidence is also the backbone of the evidence that the sickle cell gene evolved as a protection against P. falciparum malaria

The second line of evidence comes from directly comparing the level of parasitaemia in normal and G6PD deficient heterozygote females. This was found to be significantly lower in the heterozygotes than in normal females. The G6PD heterozygotes are females whose red blood cells are a mixture of normal and deficient cells. Thirdly, at the cellular level, Professor Lucio Luzzatto and his colleagues at the University of Ibadan, College of Medicine, compared the rate of parasitization of normal and G6PD deficient erythrocytes within the blood of heterozygote females, and found that normal erythrocytes consistently had more parasites than deficient erythrocytes.[126]

These results point to a likelihood of a G6PD enzyme deficiency being responsible for protection against P. falciparum malaria, but the mechanism of that protection is not fully understood; for example, the female homozygotes in whose blood all the erythrocytes are G6PD deficient, are not protected. It would appear therefore that the protection is not a direct function of enzyme deficiency. The Ibadan group has proposed that the protective effect of G6PD deficiency comes from the presence in the heterozygote, of the mosaic of both

---

[126] L. Luzzatto, O Sodeinde & G. Martini, Genetic variation in the host and adaptive phenomena in Plasmodium falciparum infection, p. 159-173. in: Malaria and the Red Cell (London, Pitman,1983).

G6PD deficient and normal erythrocytes. The parasite can adapt in a situation where all the erythrocytes are G6PD deficient, by making its own variant of G6PD enzyme; but it cannot adapt in the heterozygote where there is a mosaic of deficient and normal red blood cells. Since the parasite cannot develop without the G6PD enzyme, the heterozygote is partially protected from Plasmodium falciparum malaria.

This must not be regarded as the last word on the mechanism by which G6PD deficiency partially protects against Plasmodium falciparum malaria. It is a sad reflection of our increasing intellectual dependence on European models that emphasis on malaria research appears to be moving away from the kind of fundamental work represented by G6PD deficiency and sickle cell trait research undertaken in the 1950s to the 1970s by men like Boyo, Edozien, Luzzatto and Shodeinde, to current trends which focus on plasmodicidal drugs and insecticide-impregnated nets which in the long run actually run counter to the grain of the biological equilibrium that existed before the new trends.

iii. Sickle cell trait
Haemoglobin is a protein molecule contained within the membrane of the red blood corpuscles (rbc). It has the critically important function of transporting oxygen (which it extracts from the the air in the lungs) to the tissues of the body where the oxygen is used for various metabolic processes, and then returning the carbon dioxide produced by the tissues to the lungs for expulsion and beginning the cycle all over again. Haemoglobin is one of the wonders of creation!

The American physician Herrick (1910) first reported the presence of sickled rbcs in the blood of a West Indian medical student suffering from anaemia. He subsequently associated these peculiarly shaped enlongated rbcs with severe anaemia, that is now known to be characteristic of this form of sickle cell disorder (SCD). Sickle cell disorder refers to a group of genetic disorders that are characterized by the predominance of haemoglobin S (see below). Sickle cell disorder includes sickle cell anaemia (SS), sickle haemoglobin C disease (SC), sickle beta thalassemia plus (SB+ Thal) and other rare combinations of abnormal haemoglobins and haemoglobin S.[127]

Sickle cell anaemia, the form of sickle cell disorder most frequently encountered in Nigeria is described here as an example of this group of diseases. Some individuals in Plasmodium falciparum malaria endemic areas are born with an abnormal form of the haemoglobin molecule which, under certain circumstances, undergoes transformation causing the rbcs containing it to change from the normal discoid, to a "sickle" shape. The sickle-shaped rbcs obstruct blood flow in the capillaries that carry oxygenated blood to different organs. In the past this physical obstruction to blood flow was thought to be the main cause of the ischemia that characterizes sickle cell disorder, however, results of more recent research suggest that molecular inflammatory mechanisms contribute signifi-cantly to the condition. The sickled rbc has a tendency to adhere to capillary endothelium,

---

[127] For more details see chapter 14, D.T. Okpako, Principles of Pharmacology. A tropical approach, 2nd ed. (Cambridge University press, 2003).

thereby triggering the release of pro-inflammatory cytokines and a cascade of inflammatory reactions. This has led to the suggestion that when an SS person has a crisis it should be recognized as an inflammatory disease.[128]

Inheritance of haemoglobin S

The abnormal haemoglobin is termed haemoglobin S (Hb-S) while the normal molecule is haemoglobin A (Hb-A). Haemoglobin types are inherited by Mendelian mechanisms: An individual who inherits identical sickle cell genes from both parents is a sickle-cell homozygote (Hb-SS) and usually suffers from sickle cell disorder. Most of the haemoglobin in his red blood cells is Hb-S. An individual who inherits normal haemoglobin genes from both parents is a normal homozygote (Hb-AA); but if the child inherits Hb-S from one parent and Hb-A from the other, she/he is heterozygote (Hb-AS). About 25-40% of the haemoglobin in a heterozygote is Hb-S. This amount of Hb-S is not enough to cause sickling under normal circumstances. The heterozygote thus has the sickle cell trait but does not suffer sickle cell disease. Such an individual is a carrier of the sickle cell gene. However, a sickle cell crisis can occur in the heterozygote at high altitudes, where the oxygen pressure is low e,g., high mountains, or aircraft flying at very high altitudes. Importantly, the Hb-AS person is partially protected from Plasmodium falciparum malaria. Studies show that Hb-AS children are nearly 30% protected (i.e. they are

---

[128] Jack R Lancaster, Sickle cell disease: loss of the blood's WD40. Trends in Pharmacological Sciences 2003, 24 (8): 389-391.

30% less likely to suffer from malaria than Hb-AA or Hb-SS children), and when they suffer a malaria attack, it is less severe than the malaria disease in Hb-AA or Hb-SS children.

According to A.F. Fleming, formerly a professor of haematology at Ahmadu Bello University, Zaria, and one time president of the Nigerian Sickle Cell Society, "the consequences of partial protection against intense P. falciparum parasitaemia is shown most clearly by the almost complete absence of Hb-AS children from among those dying of cerebral malaria".[129] Cerebral malaria is the fatal stage of the disease when more than about 5% of the rbcs are infected by Plasmodium falciparum.

Because malaria parasites can be seen in large numbers in the brains of those dying of cerebral malaria at autopsy, it was thought that the obstruction of blood flow in cerebral capillary vessels caused by parasitized rbcs was the main cause of the coma preceding death. However, recent evidence indicates that the coma of cerebral malaria is caused not so much by a physical obstruction of blood flow but by the pleiotropic pro-inflammatory cytokine, tumour necrosis factor (TNF) released in response to the presence of Plasmodium falciparum.[130]

---

[129] A.F. Fleming, Sickle-cell trait. genetic counseling, in: Sickle Cell Disease, a handbook for the general clinician, A.F. Fleming, editor (Churchill Livingstone, London, 1982) p. 24.

[130] See the review by I. A.Clark et al in Cytokin and Growth Factor Reviews 2006; I.A. Clark and K.A. Rockett, Nitric oxide and parasitic disease, Advances in Parasitology, 1996, (37).

Breast milk

The human infant is most vulnerable to malaria and other infectious diseases during the first few months of life when its immune system is developing. The infant at that stage is protected against infectious agents by the mother's antibodies which the infant absorbs through the placenta in utero, and after birth from breast milk. Importantly, although breast milk contains all the nutrients required for the infant's growth, it is deficient in an essential metabolite, para-aminobenzoic acid (PABA), which infectious microorganisms (malaria parasites and bacteria) need as a substrate from which to manufacture their own folic acid for growth. Microorganisms do not make PABA or they do not make enough of it, but they need it as a substrate for the manufacturing of folic acid that is essential for their growth. The human also does not manufacture PABA being an essential constituent of the normal diet. This means that an infant fed exclusively on breast milk for at least the first six months of life would be resistant to malaria infection. The parasite that invades the rbcs of such an infant cannot develop to cause disease.

Actually, this is the basic principle on which the well known anti-malaria drugs called anti-metabolites or anti-folates, e.g., pyrimethamine (Sunday-Sunday medicine!), proguanil, sulpha-doxine, fansidar etc, were formulated. These drugs have molecular structures similar to PABA and can clog up the malaria parasite's machinery in the production of folic acid from PABA. In other words, exclusive feeding of the human infant on breast milk during its most vulnerable years is the ideal anti-malaria prophylactic.

The scientific evidence that animals fed exclusively on milk are protected from malaria has been available in the medical literature since the early 1950s when Brian Maegraith first proposed that PABA is a growth factor for the malaria parasite and more recently supported by studies showing that the protection of African infants from malaria infection is not due to maternal antibodies but PABA deficiency, and confirmed in studies in rodent malaria that the parasite requires exogenous PABA for survival.

Breastfeeding is good for the general health of the infant; but because malaria is a major killer of African children under the age of 5, when the child's immune system is still developing, breastfeeding for the infant should be pointedly promoted as a means of protecting the infant from malaria. Mothers are most likely to take breastfeeding seriously if they know that this practice would protect their children from malaria.

We conclude this brief survey of partial immunity to malaria in the Africans living in endemic areas by repeating that the African child is born into this world equipped to cope with malaria, given all the protective adaptations with which he is endowed. The Creator has prepared her/him for life in a malaria endemic environment. But if the infant, from the moment of birth, is subjected to unhealthy surroundings, forced to drink water not suitable for human consumption, fed on 'cow milk formulas' instead of the mother's breast milk and becomes overwhelmed by infections against which the child has no natural protection and the child dies before the age of five, it is naïve to blame it all on malaria.

This is not to deny the significant health risk that the malaria disease represents and the need to eradicate it from tropical Africa. The necessity for its eradication is an urgent matter in the interest of all humanity. Global warming and people migration are threatening to spread malaria-infected anopheles mosquitoes to parts of the world where malaria was once endemic including parts of Europe. Re-emergence of malaria in such places where the people have lost all natural resistance to the disease could spell health disaster of a greater magnitude than we are now seeing in Africa. Therefore, any strategy designed to eradicate or substantially reduce the burden of malaria parasites in Africa, is an important strategy for reasons other than health reasons. The fear of malaria which prevented significant numbers of Europeans and non-immune people from settling in West Africa in the 19th and 20th centuries, is also now impeding economic development and free movement of people to and from West Africa in the 21st century; and, underpinning the draconian visa and immigration requirements for entry into Euro-American countries, is the fear that West Africans carrying malaria parasites in their blood or infected female anopheles mosquitoes in their agbada folds may re-establish malaria in the countries from which it had been eradicated. Sub-Saharan Africa is the main reservoir from which the disease can be reintroduced into Europe. So for compelling reasons malaria must be eradicated, but that is a long-term programme. The most promising strategy in that regard is immunization which is proving to be a daunting scientific problem. In the meantime every effort must be directed at finding affordable preventive and curative measures to save the most vulnerable subsets of the African population from the disease.

The role of the WHO

The African child comes into this world endowed with an adequate survival kit, so that with political will and mobilization of local resources, a lot can be done by African governments to supplement the infant's natural endowments and thereby change the statistics on infant mortality in Africa. The WHO, the world's technical committee on health should not, inadvertently, give the impression to African governments, some of whom do not always show that they have the keenest sense of responsibility to their people, that the problems of high infant mortality are straightforward technical/medical problems to be solved with a drug or insecticide impregnated mosquito nets, thereby letting African leaders off the hook of responsibility, to provide essential social services including potable water to every household. WHO and other development partners involved in the malaria control project know this. We urge that, whenever the opportunity arises, they should emphasize that the good anti-malaria drug or insecticide-impregnated nets which they recommend and supply, are not substitutes for the hard work of governments to provide basic infrastructure necessary to lift the people out of poverty.

Chapter 16

Treatment of Fever in Traditional African Medicine

T he treatment of illness with plant remedies is an important part of the history of medicine. Human beings in every place and culture, without scientific evidence, many times over, came to the knowledge of the essential plants for the treatment of the ailment from which the people most regularly suffered. For example, ancient Europeans discovered Salix alba (willow) for the treatment of rheumatoid arthritis, a disease from which Europeans suffered frequently in their severely cold climates at a time when suitable clothing and efficient heating systems had not been developed, and at a time when neither the plant's phytochemistry nor the cause of rheumatoid arthritis was known. More than 100 years elapsed before the glycoside salicin, from which acetylsalicylic acid (aspirin) was eventually synthesized, was isolated from the willow bark. And, it was not until 1971 that John Vane showed that aspirin cures fever, aches and pains by an anti-inflammatory action which involves the inhibition of prostaglandin synthesis. He was awarded the 1982 Nobel Prize in medicine for this discovery, and knighted Sir John by the Queen of England.

But as it often happens with pharmacology we have not heard the last word on the mechanism of action of the willow bark; for it has now emerged from recent studies that flavonoids and polyphenols may contribute more to the potent anti-inflammatory and analgesic effects of the crude willow bark than salicin.[131] These compounds are widely distributed in the plant kingdom and have been identified in the plants frequently used as traditional medicines for the treatment of common ailments as already pointed out.

Other examples of prescience medicinal plant discoveries by ancient man in different parts of the world include Cinchona (the source of quinine), Artemisia (the source of artemisinin), Rauvolfia (the source of reserpine), Digitalis (the source of digoxin). The Nigerian variety of Rauvolfia, R. vomitoria has been used for the treatment of psychosis in traditional medicine in different parts of Nigeria since ancient times. In Nigeria where witchcraft has been viewed as an evil supernatural force from ancient times, the people came to the knowledge of numerous plants for use as ordeal poisons in witchcraft detection. The best known example is the esere bean – Physostigma venenosum (for the source of physostigmine (see pages 169-171).

Fever, aches and pains
Fever, aches and pains are the commonest symptoms of illness known to man and indigenous African people must have experienced and treated these symptoms

---

[131] J. Vlachojannis, F. Magora, S. Chrubasik, Willow species and aspirin: different mechanisms of action, Phytotherapy and Research 2011 (25): 1102-1104.

regularly with commonly known plant remedies as we have indicated in Part 2 of the book. In African medicine, traditional healers and indigenous people make a distinction between chronic life-threatening illness of unknown cause which I have referred to simply as serious illness, for which treatment requires esoteric consultations including divination, incantations and sacrifices and, minor ailments which can be treated with commonly known plant remedies. The point being stressed here is that fever, aches and pains were of such frequent occurrence in traditional African societies, that the people came, by some intuitive means as was the historical experience of people the world over, to the knowledge of plant remedies for these symptoms of unwellness.

The other reason why particular attention has to be paid to fever in any discussion of herbal treatment in African medicine is this: One of the features that distinguishes TAM from modern medicine is the availability of the latter to modern technology for diagnosis of diseases of internal organs. In TAM fever is the one symptom of a probable internal ailment that can be identified accurately without the application of technology. And, fever is the quintessential manifestation of inflammation, a biological complex mechanism that underlies the pathology of many diseases including malaria.

Fever is the most important universally recognized indicator of unwellness known to humanity. Shortly after I married Kath, a Welsh woman from Caernarvon, North Wales, in September 1967, on a day when I felt out of sorts, she asked in a concerned tone of voice, "Are you not well?"—while simultaneously placing her palm on my forehead, exactly as my late mother, Obien, an Ughievwen woman from Erhuwaren in Delta State, Nigeria, would have done, to see if I had a fever.

People in traditional African societies knew and treated fever (whatever its cause) frequently. Despite the absence of empirical data to that effect, one can cite the following grounds for believing that the traditional African treatment of fever with plant remedies was as effective as expected of any treatment.

i.   Fever can be diagnosed without a thermometer

It is common knowledge that raised body temperature is a sign of illness. If the body temperature of the baby on the mother's back, skin-to-skin, goes up by a fraction of a degree, the mother knows that something is wrong. In many instances of infection, the body temperature of the ill person is higher than that of a normal person. This is true diagnosis, based as diagnosis should be, on the difference between a normal value and the value in the ill person. What is being emphasized here is that fever is one symptom of illness that indigenous people indisputably recognized. One could not ask, 'How did they diagnose fever?' as one might reasonably ask, 'How did they determine raised blood pressure, high blood sugar or a failing heart?' Indigenous people could not diagnose these latter problems with assurance, because they lacked the appropriate technologies which are now available in modern medicine, but they could diagnose fever! Plants that are effective in the treatment of fever are thus widely known in Nigerian rural and urban communities. The people regularly use these anti-fever remedies. If a traditional healer from any part of Nigeria were to point to a plant as an effective anti-fever remedy, you better believe it! Whereas if he claims to be able to cure hypertension permanently, you have to wonder, as the University of Ibadan hypertension specialist Professor Emeritus Akinkugbe reminds us, 'How does he measure blood pressure'?[132] We can assume that fever due to malaria or other infections, must have occurred frequently among traditional populations; the people in a given community appear to use the same plants repeatedly for its treatment; they would not if the remedies did not work (see pages 122-123 for an example I cited earlier, Phyllanthus amarus).

ii. Traditional anti-fever plant remedies possess anti-inflammatory properties

The other ground we can cite as circumstantial evidence that plant remedies used in traditional African societies to treat fever were effective is this: Scientific analyses of some of these plants show that their aqueous or alcoholic extracts possess anti-inflammatory properties in various experimental models. The most famous of these methods is the rat paw oedema model. In this experiment a small volume of an inflammation producing agent such as carageenan is injected subcutaneously in the the rat's hindpaw. This causes a swelling similar to the swelling in the joints of an arthritic human patient. An anti-

---

[132] Here Professor O.O.Akinkugbe tells the story of his encounter (at a conference in 1976) with a tall distinguished-looking octogenarian herbalist from Ouagadougou, who gave a dissertation on the management of high blood pressure. After his talk, I had the temerity to ask the fundamental question: "How did you measure the blood pressure?" The answer was prompt and short— "You are a young man."

inflammatory plant extract or drug administered to the rat, orally or subcutaneously, prior to the carrageenan injection reduces the inflammation and the swelling. Pharmacologists have devised many methods for measuring the size of the swelling and hence the degree of inflammation and the effect of anti-inflammatory drug or plant extract. This model is widely used for determining whether a new drug or plant extract has anti-infammatory properties and therefore its potential as treatment of rheumatoid arthritis. Nigerian scientists employing this and other methods have demonstrated that many commonly used anti-fever remedies known to local communities possess demonstrable anti-inflammatory properties. This is indirect evidence that when such plants produce clinical relief from fever, they do so by suppressing inflammation.

The concoction famously called agbo (in Yoruba) is an aqueous/alcoholic extract of leaves and the bark of plants such as Morinda lucida (oruwo), Azadirachta indica (dogonyaro), Magnifera indica (mango) and Carica papaya (pawpaw). Agbo is used to treat fever, aches and pains. The Urhobo equivalent of agbo is uhunvwun; it consists of roots and barks of medicinal plants macerated in ogogoro (locally brewed gin), palm wine or water and taken to ward off fever, aches and pains. The demonstration that extracts from many of these plants have anti-inflammatory properties is proof of principle. Fever is the human body's characteristic expression of inflammation (see O.A. Olajide for references to publications on Nigerian plants with anti-inflammatory properties).[133] Inflammation processes cause the release of prostaglandins which interfere with the temperature regulation mechanisms in the hypothalamus and a rise in body temperature.

It is, therefore, safe to conclude that traditional African societies knew plants that could be used for the treatment of fever. In Nigeria such plants are a common knowledge in many communities. There is, therefore, an urgent need to explore the anti-inflammatory mechanisms of action of these plants in detail. This is an area of research in which Nigerian scientists should seek to seriously develop research capacity, with the real possibility of original discovery of important medicines. Traditional African communities seem to have done the basic screening of local plants with significant anti-fever properties, and fever is the body's response to inflammation which now appears to be a major component of the pathology of malaria and many other diseases.

Fever and malaria infection

In Nigeria the term malaria is frequently used synonymously with fever; often, without blood smear confirmation; fever is self-diagnosed and then self-medicated with anti-malaria drugs as if it is malaria disease. This is because of the general experience that the commonest most consistent symptom of malaria infection is fever. Not all fever is malaria fever of course, but if someone has acute incapacitating fever, aches and

---

[133] For a comprehensive list of such publications see: www.2.hud. ac.uk/sas/—/profile.php?sata. . .

pains anywhere in Nigeria, there is a high probability that the cause is malaria. A corollary to this assumption is made by Nigerian scientists who are searching for anti-malarial drugs in local plants, namely, that traditional anti-fever remedies are anti-malarial, i.e., that they must contain plasmodicidal chemicals that kill the plasmodium malaria parasites. Such an assumption is based on the experience that all currently available anti-malaria drugs are plasmodicidal. So, what usually happens with this research approach is that if the plant extract does not reveal a chemical entity with specific plasmodicidal property, the matter is, unfortunately, not pursued further. The overarching paradigm in conventional malaria research compels the search for a drug that is selectively toxic to the parasite at a dose that is safe in the human. The idea that a plant with anti-inflammatory, but no specific plasmodicidal properties, may be useful therapy in the partially immune African has never been considered as a serious proposition.

A common finding from current research is that many of the plant remedies used widely in Nigeria have anti-inflammatory properties, but to date there is no consistent evidence that the effectiveness of these plants can be attributed to chemical entities with specific plasmodicidal properties. Since these plant remedies are effective in controlling fever, and fever is a characteristic expression of inflammation, we conclude that the plants' effectiveness in suppressing fever is due to their anti-inflammatory activities. Since malaria is endemic in these communities, is also relatively safe to conclude that in many cases the fever is caused by malaria and that the treatment of fever was an effective symptomatic treatment of malaria in the partially immune African. Therefore we make the following unproven but circumstantially plausible and testable hypothesis:

> The clinical benefits of traditional plant remedies used in the treatment of malaria/fever can be attributed to their anti-inflammatory properties; for most adult Africans who are partially immune to malaria, it is enough to treat the plasmodium-induced inflammation, and the subsequent surge in immune activity would eliminate the parasites in this category of patients.

If this idea proves to be correct, it would mean that there existed in traditional African societies, an effective malaria treatment strategy that avoided direct drug attack on the malaria parasite and which at the same time enabled the individual's immunity to be reinforced against the parasite during repeated exposures to the infection. We now know that it is the direct attack on the parasite in an attempt to kill it, in modern chemotherapy that resulted in the emergence of chloroquine resistance and now multi-drug resistant malaria. Also, elimination of the parasite with drugs weakens the individual's resistance to malaria infection.

What this means is that malaria infection in the partially immune adult African was not, and need not be a serious life threatening illness. This would imply that an effective treatment of malaria-induced inflammation is a cure for malaria in partially immune Africans, not a mere symptomatic treatment. The historical evidence that Africa was not decimated by malaria before the advent of the new chemotherapy, points to the probability that indigenous African people survived the deadly parasite because of a combination of partial immunity and the availability of effective herbal treatments.

In concluding this section let me stress that the hypothesis does not imply that every case of malaria can be cured with aspirin. The theory is applicable to large numbers of adult Africans living in malaria endemic areas who are partially immune to the disease as described above but may not necessarily apply to subsets of the population such as people in the extremes of age (infants and the elderly), pregnant women and people living with HIV/AIDS and TB whose immunity may be compromised, and it would not apply to naïve non-immune people visiting, or resident in malaria endemic areas. But, because the theory applies to an overwhelmingly large number of resident Africans, I think it would be well worth putting it to the test. And, the idea that a large number of otherwise healthy African adults are semi-immune to malaria ought to be an important factor in any scheme designed for the judicious use of expensive plasmodicidal anti-malaria drugs. Not every one who has fever should have to take such drugs (see chapter 17).

Inflammation is a complex phenomenon involving different mechanisms. The critical mechanism in one disease may be quite different from that in another disease. The theory should therefore not be interpreted simplistically to imply, for example, that nonsteroidal anti-inflammatory drugs such as aspirin or ibuprofen would cure malaria in the partially immune person. That would be wrong: NSAIDs of the asprin type act by inhibiting cyclooxygenase (COX) enzymes. But as can be seen from the review of mechanisms of the anti-inflammatory action of herbal extracts in the appendix 2, herbal remedies contain a cocktail of substances that can produce an anti-inflammatory action by many different mechanisms e.g., antioxidant activities, inhibition of lipoxygenase and inducible nitric oxide synthase, enzymes catalyzing the formation of pro-inflammatory cytokines and nuclear transcription activating factor (NF-kB), etc. Herbal remedies therefore represent a more likely source of the range of chemical entities acting together to inhibit the array of mechanisms underlying inflammation in malaria.

Chapter 17

Inflammation and Malaria

I n the last two chapters I have tried to make the case that herbal remedies were successful in the treatment of malaria in partially immune Africans, not because the remedies were plasmodicidal, but because they possessed anti-inflammatory properties. In a remarkable convergence of ancient intuition and new science, recent researches now reveal that malaria disease is indeed, fundamentally, an inflammatory disease.

Let me therefore devote the following pages to a historical survey of the evidence that inflammation mechanisms are an important component of the pathology, not only of malaria, but also of many other chronic diseases of man. The late Professor Brian Maegraith observed[134] that in cerebral malaria-induced coma, an infusion of quinine or chloroquine may rapidly restore the patient to consciousness, before the drugs had killed the parasites causing the disease. The initial rapid relief he predicted, was due to an anti-inflammatory action of chloroquine. Later, Maegraith and his Nigerian student, the late Professor Ayodele Tella demonstrated that in the Rhesus monkey, malaria infection was accompanied by a

---

[134] Brian Maegraith, Pathological Processes in Malaria and Black Water Fever (Oxford, Scientific Publications, 1948) p. 367.

rise in plasma levels of bradykinin, a powerful pleiotropic mediator of inflammation.

Over the years, Maegraith's hypothesis that inflammation is a major underlying mechanism contributing to the pathology of malaria has been supported by the results of basic biomedical research worldwide. Even the common clinical experience with chloroquine—a drug with significant anti-inflammatory properties—supports the hypothesis. With chloroquine, a resolution of clinical symptoms is relatively rapid following the usual dosage regimen, whereas with drugs such as fansidar, halofanthrine, artemisinin, etc, which, though plasmodicidal, lack significant anti-inflammatory properties, relief from clinical symptoms is slower, usually necessitating the additional use of a non-steroidal anti-inflammatory drug such as aspirin or paracetamol.

Cytokine theory of malaria

Ian Clark and his colleagues at the Australian National Uni versity, Canberra, Australia, have in the past decades, amassed impressive evidence for the role of inflammation in malaria. They demonstrated [135] that there was a highly significant positive correlation between plasma concentrations of the pro-inflammatory cytokine, tumour necrosis factor (TNF) and parasitaemia, in Plasmodium falciparum malaria disease in children. The theory is that the presence of malaria parasites in red blood corpuscles (rbcs) increases their tendency to adhere to capillary endothelium. Adhesion of rbcs to endothelium is the

---

[135] I.A. Clark, K.A.Rockett andW.B. Cowden Ann Trop Med Parasitol 1996 (90): 395-402.

trigger for a casacade of inflammatory mechanisms which characterize malaria disease, e.g., activation of induced nitric oxide synthase (iNOS) to produce high inflammatory (nanomole) quantities of nitric oxide. Normally, the endothelium generates low anti-inflammatory (picomole) amounts of nitric oxide which, with prostacyclin, prevent rbcs adhesion to the capillary endothelium; rbcs adhesion also leads to the production of high amounts of the proinflammatory cytokine, TNF which in low concentrations would normally inhibit parasite growth for host defence, but the cytokine becomes harmful to the host in high concentrations. A comprehensive review of more than three hundred original research publications[136] shows that what is now called the cytokine theory applies to acute infectious diseases in general including typhoid, sepsis, influenza, vivax and falciparum malaria. Pro-inflammatory cytokines such as tumour necrosis factor (TNF) and interleukin-1 (Il-1) are the critical mechanisms by which systemic disease is amplified in these infections. But there is a lot yet to be understood about the complex inflammatory mechanisms in malaria disease.

The raised level of proinflammatory cytokines and other inflammation mediators in the plasma of infected patients is the most likely explanation for the symptoms of acute infectious disease—anorexia, tiredness, aching joints and muscles, fever, sleepiness etc. that patients experience. The hypoxia and metabolic acidosis seen in severe malaria is caused, not by vascular sequestration of

[136] Ian Clark, Alison C. Budd, Lisa M Alleva,and William B. Cowden, Human malaria disease: a consequence of inflammatory cytokine release, Malaria Journal 2006 (5): 85.

parasitized red blood cells as previously assumed, but by TNF-mediated mitochondrial shut down.

Fever is a key indicator of illness, and has long been postulated that an endogenous fever regulator must exist. It now seems that interleukin 1 (IL-1), one of the prototype proinflammatory cytokines, is the endogenous pyrogen.[137] Cytokines released into the peripheral circulation as a result of bacterial or parasitic infection, can enter the brain and affect the temperature regulating mechanism in the hypothalamus; cytokines can also stimulate the production of PGE2, a highly potent pyrogen, in the brain.

The inflammatory mechanisms contributing to malaria pathology are complex and not yet fully understood. Hence the call in this book (see pg 306, chapter 19) for the establishment of a well funded centre for the study of inflammation and malaria in Nigeria. What the available evidence suggests is that inflammation is a critically important component of malaria disease, and it would appear that in the partially immune African adult suffering from malaria, effective amelioration of the inflammation associated with the disease is a cure of the disease; the immune system in the partially immune person is sufficiently alert to eliminate the parasite, once the inflammation mechanisms are suppressed.

Traditional herbal treatment of malaria was a remarkably appropriate strategy

It is intriguing that African ancients fortuitously evolved herbal treatments for malaria/fever which consisted of

---

[137] B. Contri, I. Tabarean, C. Andrei and T. Bafai, Cytokines and fever, Frontiers in Bioscience 2004 (9): 1433-1449.

plants with anti-inflammatory properties; in the light of the new research, the indigenous Africans' treatment strategy can now be appreciated as most appropriate for the partially immune who are continuously exposed to malaria in endemic areas.

A treatment strategy directed at ameliorating the malaria pathology rather than killing the parasite may seem at first sight to be worthless, as being a 'merely' symptomatic treatment. The symptoms must return if the cause, that is the malaria parasite, is not eliminated. That is the thinking in modern malaria chemotherapy where the objective is to attack the parasite, so as to selectively kill it or prevent its growth. The proposal here is that effective treatment of the symptoms in the partially immune person is tantamount to cure. This traditional way of dealing with malaria has advantages when compared to the modern chemotherapeutic approach that is based on the use of plasmodicidal anti-malaria drugs. In the first place, treatment of malaria-induced pathology enables the immune system of the partially immune person to be mobilized against the parasite by activating already primed immune mechanisms, as can be inferred from earlier studies;[138] in this way the immune capacity of the individual to deal with further infections is reinforced. On the other hand, as can be inferred also from earlier research findings by Edozien, Boyo & Morley[139] plasmodicidal chemotherapy produces the opposite effect,

---

[138] J.C Edozien, The serum proteins of healthy adult Nigerians. Journal of Clinical Pathology 1957,10(3): 276-279.

[139] J.C.Edozien, A.E.Boyo, and D.C. Morley, The relationship of serum gamma-globulin concentration to malaria and sickling. Journal of Clinical Pathology 1960 (13): 118-123.

namely, it dampens the immune capacity of the partially immune to resist malaria infection. Furthermore, experience from the use of plasmo-dicidal anti-malaria drugs since the inception of modern chemotherapy, is that parasite resistance to these drugs soon develops. Drug resistance is the parasite's response to attempts at eliminating it.

It may help to briefly explain here how resistance develops to plasmodicidal anti-malaria drugs. In any given population of malaria parasites there are varying degrees of sensitivity to the killing effect of a plasmodicidal drug. The drug kills the most sensitive species in the parasite population, but less sensitive members survive, giving rise eventually to a new population of parasites that is resistant to the killing effect of the anti-malaria drug. Malaria treatment that focuses on the inflammation component of the disease achieves two things:

i. it allows the partially immune person's immunological defences against malaria to be reinforced after every bout of infection, and

ii. it avoids inciting the parasite into mobilizing its considerable arsenal of resistance mechanisms.

The traditional African treatment of malaria has parallels in modern chemotherapy

The indigenous Africans peoples' treatment of malaria which targets the pathology rather than the plasmodium is an approach that is worthy of serious consideration and further research. It is not a frivolous idea but one that has parallels in the use of bacteriostatic and bactericidal antibiotics in the treatment of bacterial infections in modern medicine. In the latter system we quite often use selectively acting agents, such as sulphonamides, designed to inhibit the growth of the causative organism. These so called bacteriostatic agents do not kill the bacteria, whereas antibiotics such as penicillin that kill the bacteria are bactericidal agents. The bacteriostatic agents cure the infection because the ill person's immune system overcomes and eliminates the non-growing population of the pathogen.

What one is saying with respect to indigenous treatment of malaria is not too dissimilar to the scenario in the use of bacteriostatic agents in modern medicine. In the African living continuously in a malaria endemic environment, partial immunity to malaria provides a unique background in which anti-fever/anti-inflammatory herbal remedies act like bacterio-static agents.

Inflammation is a common factor in the pathology of many diseases

Inflammation is defined by the Chambers Science and Technology Dictionary as "the reaction of a living tissue to injury or infection, the affected part becoming red, hot, painful and swollen, due to hyperaemia, exudation of lymph, and escape into the tissue of blood cells".

This definition takes off from Lewis's classic triple response which is widely recognized as the skin reaction (clearly observable in a white person's skin) following an insect bite or subcutaneous injection of histamine. Inflammation can follow bacterial, viral, parasitic infection or allergen/IgE antibody reaction occurring in internal organs. The response consists of complex processes initially as a defence mechanism. Through symptoms such as aches, pains, fever etc, caused by mediators of the inflammation reaction, the attention of the person experiencing the injury is drawn to the problem. But the biological activities of these mediators such as pro-inflammatory cytokines and prostaglandins in high concentrations are known causes of illness.

Well known examples of inflammation diseases are rheumatoid arthritis, inflammatory bowel disease, asthma, colitis. Malaria has, of recent, been understood to be an inflammatory disease mainly because, contrary to traditional scientific belief, the major cause of illness is not the parasite itself but numerous pro-inflammatory agents released by the host due to the presence of the parasite. The symptoms of the disease are due to the biological activities of these pro-inflammatory mediators.

The findings from different laboratories worldwide that inflammation mechanisms contribute significantly, not only to malaria, but also to the pathology of many other important diseases should be of particular interest to the African medical scientist. One observation that has baffled researchers in African medicine for years is the claim by traditional healers that one plant remedy can be a cure for different diseases, often with contradictory pathological manifestations.[140] Can anti-inflammatory properties in these plants explain the diverse uses of the same plant in traditional African medicine?

The fact that many Nigerian medicinal plant extracts have been shown to possess anti-inflammatory properties is a compelling reason why we should focus research on the detailed mechanism of action of these plants, bearing in mind that inflammatory mechanisms are complex and

---

[140] See the study on the plant Crotolaria retusa, (Koropo by Una Maclean referred to on page 204 and comments by Professor Shellard on pages 199 and 203.

differ from one disease to another, and plant products affect inflammation by different mechanisms. Specific inflammation mechanisms and therefore anti-inflammatory drug targets differ from one disease to another. That is why although asthma and rheumatoid arthritis are inflammatory diseases, aspirin or drugs like it can be used to treat arthritis but are contraindicated in asthma. This understanding has intensified the search for anti-inflammatory drugs with different modes of action, and attention has particularly focused on plants as potential sources of anti-inflammatory medicines worldwide[141] see also the review by Nworu & Akah in appendix 2 (pp. 329-358). Let us briefly sketch the inflammation mechanisms underlying the pathology of some major diseases.

i. Asthma

Until about 40 years ago, asthma was thought to be simply a Type 1 Hypersensitivity Reaction in which an allergen interacted with IgE antibodies that were fixed to mast cells in the bronchioles. It was believed that histamine and other mediators released as a result of such antigen-antibody reaction caused the characteristic bronchoconstriction or narrowing of the airways and difficulty in breathing, that are common outward manifestations of the disease. This was why the sensitized guinea-pig which responds characteristically with bronchospasm on challenge with a sensitizing antigen was employed as an animal model for the study of asthma in many laboratories. That view is now known to be an

---

[141] A. A. Izzo and F. Capasso, Herbal medicine, cancer prevention and cyclooxygenase 2 inhibition. Trends in Pharmacological Sciences 2003; (24): 218 - 219.

oversimplification. Not every asthmatic attack is due to antigen-antibody interaction. Asthma is now recognized as an inflammatory disease. The hyper-sensitivity of the bronchial muscle to constrictor agents is due to the destruction of the bronchial epithelium by cellular (leucocytes, eosinophils) and chemical (eicosanoids, nitric oxide) mediators of inflammation.[142] The result is bronchospasm which, in the asthmatic, can be caused by a variety of unrelated agents (including cold air). Bronchospasm is the defining feature of asthma and the most effective anti-asthmatic drugs are ß2-agonist bronchodilators (which also possess anti-inflammatory properties) and anti-inflammatory corticosteroids. Attempts have also been made to develop anti-asthmatic drugs that target inflammatory mediators such as leucotriene receptors. Now, new evidence[143] point to nitric oxide (NO) as playing a critical role in asthma pathology, thereby adding to the repertoire of possible inflammation-related targets for the development of anti-asthmatic drugs.

ii. Cancer

It is now well known that prostaglandins play a crucial role in cancer. The prostaglandin synthase enzymes, fatty acid cyclooxygenases (COXs) are over-expressed in many different types of cancer. As in inflammation in general, cyclooxygenase-2 (COX-2) appears to be the dominant

---

[142] See for example P.J. Barnes, Pathophysiology of asthma, British Journal of Clinical Pharmacology 1996 42 (1): 3-10.

[143] Reviewed by H. Meurs, Maaarsingh and J. Zaagsma, Arginase and asthma: novel insights into nitirc oxide homeostasis and airway hyper-responsiveness, Trends in Pharmacological Sciences 2003 (24): 450-455.

enzyme responsible for the production of prostaglandin E-2 in cancer. PGE-2 contributes to tumour development and growth by different mechanisms. The list of malignant conditions in which there is now overwhelming evidence for a crucial role for COX-2 is long and includes cancers of the colon, stomach, liver, pancreas, lung, breast, bladder and skin. Some selective COX-2 inhibitors have undergone clinical trials for cancer treatment as adjunct therapy with good outcome, but cardiovascular side effects of selective COX-2 inhibitors have prevented further development along these lines.

In Ibadan, more than three decades before the role of COX-2 in cancer was recognized, we reported that biopsies of the childhood tumour, Burkitt's lymphoma commonly seen in Ibadan, contains large amounts of biologically active lipids that have a similar bioassay and chromatographic characteristics to prostaglandin E2.[144] It thus seems that in this tropical tumour too, there may be an over-expression of COX enzymes, but direct evidence that COX-2 is over-expressed in Burkitt's lymphoma has not been provided, nor is there yet evidence that a judicious combination of COX-2 inhibitors with conventional chemotherapy will be of benefit in the treatment of this tumour. For more on the role of inflammation in the pathogenesis of cancer, see the review by Subbaramaiah & Dannenberg. [145]

---

[144] O.O. Ajayi and D.T. Okpako, Prostaglandin-like substances in Burkitt lymphoma tissue, Br. J. Cancer 1977 (36): 149.

[145] K. Subbaramaiah and A.J. Dannenberg, Cyclooxygenase 2: a molecular target for cancer prevention and treatment, Trends in Pharmacological Sciences 2003 (24): 96-102.

iii. Sickle cell disease

Sickle cell disease (SCD) is one of a group of genetic disorders characterized by the preponderance of an abnormal haemoglobin called haemoglobin S (HbS) in the red blood cells of the sufferer. Haemoglobin S contains the amino-acid valine instead of glutamic acid in position 6 of the beta chain of normal haemoglobin A (HbA). The abnormal haemoglobin (HbS) may polymerize in conditions of low oxygen tension, resulting in the characteristic sickle-shaped red blood cells (see page 259). The disease is typified by, among other things, repeated ischaemic episodes, giving rise to severe pain especially in the joints, haemolytic anaemia and, in severe cases, stroke. Inflammation mechanisms have recently been shown to be significant underlying factors in SCD pathology.[146] It is suggested that the presence of polymerized haemoglobin in red blood cells causes the cells to adhere to capillary endothelium, leading to the activation of inducible nitric oxide synthase (iNOS) and synthesis of inflammatory concentrations of nitric oxide. This mechanism is reminiscent of malaria disease in which the presence of the plasmodium parasite in the red blood cell increases the tendency of the latter to adhere to capillary endothelium (sequestration), leading to a cascade of inflammatory reactions and disease. So, here again we must remind ourselves that in the management of a sickle cell crisis, herbal preparations were the main resource of treatment in TAM.

Malaria and sickle cell disorder: a puzzling link

---

[146] For detailed scientific evidence see J.R. Lancaster Jr, Sickle cell disease: loss of the blood's WD40? Trends in Pharmacological Sciences 2003 (24): 389-391.

There are some intriguing connections between malaria disease and sickle cell disease (SCD) that scientists working in these respective fields of research seem to ignore. First of all, both diseases are red blood corpuscle (rbc) diseases. Second, the historical evidence is that the genetic modification of the sickle haemoglobin which gives rise to SCD was triggered by the Plasmodium falciparum malaria parasite which infects rbcs. Third and very importantly, a combination of normal and sickle haemoglobin genes in an individual (Hb-AS) partially protects that individual from malaria disease, whereas an individual whose haemoglobin is predominantly sickle haemoglobin (Hb-SS), is highly susceptible to malaria disease. In fact according to pathologist Professor Ed. 'B. Atta,[147] 75% of HbSS children in rural Nigeria die of SCD before the age of 5. This incidentally, is an important confounding factor in the infant mortality statistics that are usually attributed to malaria alone. Fourth, and perhaps the most intriguing of these connections is that inflammation is an important factor in the underlying pathology of both diseases and, the rbc is the disease agent.

In both diseases, the rbc's physical characteristic is perturbed such that it now has a tendency to adhere to the endothelium of the capillary blood vessel. This is the trigger for a cascade of the inflammatory reactions that characterize both diseases. What perturbs the rbcs is the presence of a nonphysiologically 'strange' element that is not normally there i.e., a parasite in the case of malaria

---

[147] Ed. B. Atta, The pathology of sickle cell disease, in: Sickle-Cell Disease, A handbook for the general clinician, A.F. Fleming, editor (Churchill Livingstone, Edinburgh, 1982) p. 42.

and, in the case of SCD, polymerized haemoglobin. There is a fifth connection between the two diseases: The rbc perturbed by the presence of this 'nonphysiological' element, activates a membrane pump which in SCD effluxes potassium and water from the interior of the red cell, an action that initiates the polymerization of sickle haemoglobin. In malaria disease, probably the same pump effluxes plasmodicidal drugs from the interior of the infected rbcs, as a drug resistance mechanism.

Exploring these connections may reveal new insights in malaria and SCD research and it calls for a closer collaboration between sickle cell and malaria disease researchers; unlike now when the two sets of scientists work independently of each other as if on completely unrelated problems.

In concluding this section let me stress that the examples I have chosen are only a few from a large number of diseases in which inflammation mechanisms are known to contribute significantly to disease pathology, enough to emphasize the importance of this area of research in the African environment. Other important examples are the degenerative diseases of the central nervous system such as Parkinson's and Alzheimer's disease.[148]

---

[148] For review see S.Weggen, M. Rogers & J. Erikson, NSAIDs: small molecules for the prevention of Alzheimer's disease or precursors for future drug development? Trends in Pharmacological Sciences 2007 (28): 536-543.

Chapter 18

Drug Resistance in Malaria

T he indigenous African herbal treatment of malaria is directed at the disease pathology, and does not directly attack the parasite. This approach merits close examination as a treatment strategy in the partially immune person: We know from experience of chemotherapy in general that it is the direct attack on a disease-causing microorganism by a selectively toxic drug that provokes the microorganism, in self defence so to speak, into developing resistance to the treatment. The traditional approach offers a plausible explanation why drug resistance was not a confounding factor when chemotherapy with plasmodicidal drugs was first introduced as malaria treatment in Africa. This chapter expatiates on the problems posed by malaria resistance to modern drugs, and how another look at traditional herbal remedies may pave the way to finding an answer to malaria drug resistance.

Multi-drug resistance in malaria
One major problem that has dogged the use of selectively toxic agents in treatment of diseases caused by microorganisms through out the history of chemotherapy is the universal tendency of the targeted pathogen to

become resistant to the chemotherapeutic agent. Over the years scientists have ingeniously invented drugs that work by a variety of mechanisms meant to overcome drug resistance; just as ingeniously, microorganisms have responded by deploying an incredible array of resistance mechanisms previously unknown to scientists in order to survive the different killing agents. Thus multidrug resistance has become a well known troublesome phenomenon in modern medicine.

In multi-drug resistance, the pathogen develops mechanisms which enable it to survive a multitude of selectively toxic drugs that may be acting by different mechanisms; for example, the Plasmodium falciparum parasite has become resistant to chloroquine, mefloquine, sulphonamide combinations, pyrime-thamine and now artemisinin. All these drugs attack the parasite by different mechanisms. This has been the experience whether the pathogen is a virus, bacterium, fungus, cancer cell or parasite. In every case, the conventional response of the pharmaceutical industry is to introduce a new drug, hopefully to which the microorganism will not develop resistance. Another common approach is to combine drugs with different mechanisms of action, in order to confuse the pathogen's resistance mechanisms. It is a raging war between the scientist and the microorganism against infectious diseases in which the microorganism usually has the upper hand, being an ancient survivor of evolutionary battles in different chemical environments long before humans were created. It should not be a surprise that one of the most serious problems facing malaria chemotherapy today is the recurrent resistance of this ancient Plasmodium falciparum parasite to chemotherapy.

Reports of a rising incidence of malaria parasite resistance to anti-malaria drugs are worrying for various reasons: Parasite resistance to drugs poses a serious problem to the efforts being made to eliminate malaria. It sets up a cycle in which resistance leads to the mandatory introduction of another generation of more potent, and usually also more difficult to use, and more expensive drugs. All these are conditions which favour the emergence of resistance to the new drug, among low income, ill-informed populations who are liable to misuse the drug. Since the deployment of chemotherapy as the main plank of malaria control strategies in Africa, Plasmodium falciparum has developed resistance to generation after generation of anti-malaria drugs, first to chloroquine and related drugs, then to the anti-metabolite sulphonamide type drugs and now it seems, to the newest drug, artemisinin. Even more worrying is the fact that the resistant plasmodium is more virulent, more deadly than the naïve parasite with evidence that with drug resistance 'has come a doubling of malaria mortality in some parts of Africa'.[149] In other words, the disease has become more dangerous and more difficult to control since modern chemotherapy.

A common attribute of the anti-malaria drugs to which resistance has developed is their high selective toxicity for the Plasmodium falciparum parasite; that is, their

---

[149] A.S. Bell and L.C. Ranford-Cartwright. A real-time PCR assay for quantifying Plasmodium falciparum infections in the mosquito vector. Int J Parasitol 2004: 34: 795–802.

target is to kill the plasmodium parasite or to prevent its growth, which amounts to the same thing. After an examination of the pattern of plasmodium resistance to these drugs, a Nigerian group of malariologists predicted two decades ago[150] that the malaria parasite may have an innate capacity to develop resistance to any drug of this kind, however initially powerful it may be at killing it. What we are experiencing is a fulfilment of that prediction and of the inevitability that future new anti-malaria drugs of this kind will fall to parasite resistance. One promising line of research attempted by the Ibadan group was to counter the resistance. They discovered that, in vitro, a diverse group of commonly used drugs when combined with a plasmodicidal drug e.g., chloroquine, to which the plasmodium parasite is resistant, can restore the sensitivity of the plasmodium to the drug; but this approach is yet to find a wide clinical application.

At the risk of sounding apocalyptic, I must warn that we are balancing on the edge of a very dangerous chemotherapeutic cliff, at an imminent point when humanity may face a Plasmodium falciparum parasite that is resistant to every plasmodicidal anti-malaria drug produced by the pharma-ceutical industry. This warning is based on a historical experience with Mycobacterium tuberculae, the pathogen that causes tuberculosis. In the 1950s, TB could be cured by using relatively simple inexpensive drugs, for example, para-aminosalicylic acid (PAS), isoniazid (INH), streptomycin, but resistance of

[150] A. Oduola, M. J. Sowunmi, A., Milhouse, et al. Innate resistance to new anti-malarial drugs in Plasmodium falciparum from Nigeria. Am. J. Trop. Med. Hyg. 1991 (86) 123-126.

the tubercle bacillus to such drugs and to every new generation of anti-TB drug subsequently introduced finally brought us to the dangerous situation we are in now. The disease caused by certain strains of the TB bacterium (extensively resistant TB) is untreatable with any existing antibiotic, singly or in combination. This is now one of the most serious challenges in modern medicine. If we allow this experience to repeat itself with plasmodicidal anti-malaria drugs, we could end up with a super plasmodium causing a virtually incurable malaria disease. Modern chemotherapy would have fundamentally changed the plasmodium parasite with which Africans lived in biological equilibrium for millennia, to a really dangerous parasite. In adopting plasmodicidal chemotherapy as the main plank of the malaria control strategy, we must not lose sight of this danger to the African population; therefore the use of these drugs must include practices that minimize the emergence of parasite resistance to new and effective anti-malaria drugs.

What the indigenous African treatment of malaria disease suggests is that it is possible to cure the disease, in the partially protected person, without killing the parasite. This is an important insight because direct attack on the parasite with plasmodicidal drugs is the stimulus for the parasite to mobilize its considerable armoury of resistance mechanisms. We should find a way to incorporate the indigenous African approach into a focussed malaria research agenda and in the smart use of existing anti-malaria drugs.

The important points to draw from this chapter on drug resistance in malaria are

i. The Plasmodium falciparum malaria parasite is endowed with an innate capacity to become resistant to any drug designed to kill it. Consequently, the search for an effective plasmodicidal drug to which the parasite is not resistant is a continuous and possibly a losing battle, though ostensibly, a commercially very profitable pursuit.

ii. The multi-drug resistant malaria parasite is more virulent and more lethal than the naïve parasite ever was before the introduction of modern chemotherapy. It is for these reasons that it is strongly suggested that scientists carefully examine the traditional African alternative approach, that is, the treatment of the disease in the partially immune person with appropriate herbal remedies because in such people treatment of the symptoms amounted to a cure of the disease. The challenge from a strategic policy point of view is to see how this African experience can be incorporated in the clinical management of malaria disease in such a way as to increase the life span of any new useful plasmodicidal anti-malaria drugs. Some suggestions in this direction are elaborated upon in the next chapter.

Chapter 19

The Importance of an Africa-centred Approach to Malaria Control

I t is a paradox that the African person for whose benefit the malaria eradication schemes are designed is not the central focus of scientific attention in the whole process. The African person's considerable genetic and immunogenic protective endowments against malaria are not taken into consideration and the Africans' considerable experience in the treatment of malaria with herbal remedies is virtually ignored. Rather it is the parasite and the non-immune person that appear to be the main focus of scientific attention.

Obviously, it can be argued that if the insecticide-impregnated nets, insecticides, vaccines and plasmodicidal drugs succeed in reducing the burden of disease in the endemic areas thereby making these areas safe for non-immune persons, that must be to everyone's benefit including the African person, a sort of biomedical top-down policy. To a certain degree this policy has been successful in West Africa. Malaria survival outlook for Europeans and other non-immune persons is now vastly better than it was in the 19th century, when the region was tagged the "white man's grave". But the Africans who were thought to be immune to malaria then, are now at greater risk from the disease than they were then.

If the African person had been at the centre of the malaria control programme, the long-term benefit would be greater for all concerned. The fact that a large proportion of Africans have immunologic- and genetic-driven adaptations which, at least partially, protect them from malaria, should have been taken advantage of, to design smart anti-malaria drug schedules in the clinical management of the disease among African populations.

Not everyone who has fever should have to take powerful resistance-provoking plasmodicidal anti-malaria drugs. The current one drug-fits-all policy in malaria disease treatment is partly responsible for the emergence of plasmodium resistance to anti-malaria drugs and treatment failures. In this chapter I elaborate on how an Africa-centred approach to malaria control would benefit humanity as a whole, not just Africans. So, what would be the essential elements in such an approach?

Factors to consider in an Africa-centred approach
to malaria control

The Africa-inspired Roll Back Malaria (RBM) programme, sponsored by the WHO and various Western donors, is a top-down policy that fails to take into account the African experience of malaria, an ancient malady with which African people lived in biological equilibrium for millennia before European contact. Some of the WHO recommendations, e.g., the use of insecticide-impregnated mosquito nets and cheap plasmodicidal anti-malaria drugs available to all are not only unsustainable, but actually run counter to the grain of the age old equilibrium. The RBM policies are largely guided by the European fear of malaria, as they recall their peoples' experience of the disease in their fatal contact with it 500 years ago.[151] If the aim of malaria control and eradication is to benefit all humanity, it is necessary to centre the programme on the African person, and the plan should include the consideration of the following factors.

i. Partial immunity of the African

As described above already, Hb-AS and G6PD deficient individuals are partially protected from Plasmodium falciparum malaria. One practical use to which this fact can be put in the war against malaria is for every Nigerian to know his/her genotype in respect of these two genetic markers. About one quarter to one third of the Nigerian population is partially protected by these mechanisms which are in addition to the acquired immunity to malaria that all Nigerians possess. About 25-30% of a population of 160 million amounts to a very large number (40-50 million) of Nigerians with inbuilt natural protection against Plasmodium falciparum malaria disease. It should be possible to devise smart ways so that not every adult, otherwise healthy, Nigerian with 'malaria fever' should have to take a powerful plasmodicidal antimalaria drug. A large number of these partially protected Nigerians would most probably need no more than an antipyretic or a traditional herbal preparation and a few days rest to

---

[151] D.T. Okpako, Malaria and Indigenous Knowledge in Africa, (Ibadan, Ibadan University Press, 2011).

overcome their malaria fever. And very importantly, subsequent episodes will be progressively less and less likely to knock them down as their immune mechanisms are repeatedly reinforced.

There are of course other reasons why Nigerians must know their status in respect of these two genetic markers. If an Hb-AS marries an Hb-AS, the couple has 1 in 4 chance of producing an Hb-SS child who will suffer from sickle cell anaemia, and who may die before the age of 5, unless draconian health precautions are taken. It is imperative therefore that young people should have this knowledge to make an informed decision before committing themselves to marriage and raising a family. The aim of a national campaign should be to discourage marital unions between two young people each with the sickle cell gene. This should in due course reduce the sickle cell gene density in the population as a whole.

Moreover, G6PD deficient individuals are liable to suffer haemolysis if they take certain types of drugs[152] such as sulphonamides and even anti-malaria drugs. This was why Lucio Luzzatto advocated for many years that Nigerians should know their G6PD status, and doctors, pharmacists and nurses practising in this environment should be conversant with the types of drugs that can provoke adverse reactions in G6PD deficient individuals.

---

[152] L. Luzzatto, Glucose-6-phosphate-dehydrogenase and other genetic factors interacting with drugs. in: Ethnic Differences in Reaction to Drugs and Xenobiotics, Werner Kalow, H. Werner Goedde, Dharam P. Agarwal, editors (New York, Alan R. Liss, 1986).

ii. Plasmodicidal anti-malaria drugs should be 'prescription only medicines'

The fact that drug resistance is a major problem with malaria chemotherapy should be reflected in the way these drugs are prescribed and used. Pharmacists, doctors and nurses know this problem from experience of chemotherapy of bacterial and viral infections as well as cancer and the precautions usually taken to minimize the chances of drug resistance in the chemotherapy of these diseases. Even ordinary non-medical people are familiar with the concept that the misuse of chemotherapeutic agents can lead to the emergence of drug resistance and, that therefore a certain amount of control must apply to the prescription and use of, for example, antibiotics. Doctors do not prescribe an antibiotic until diagnosis establishes that the cause of disease is bacterial infection, and the patient must be instructed to complete the prescribed schedule of doses. Such control is an attempt to avoid the misuse of the drugs and thereby minimize the emergence of resistance.

In malaria chemotherapy where drug resistance is equally problematic, this principle has not been brought out strongly enough, either among doctors and pharmacists or in the general population who daily use antimalarial drugs. We should do so. New, effective plasmodicidal antimalarial drugs should be prescription-only medicines to ensure that such drugs are used only when the fever has been properly diagnosed as malaria. Self-medication with potent plasmodicidal antimalarial drugs without a doctor's prescription should be recognized as a misuse of these drugs and should be actively discouraged. It must also be emphasized that it is the misuse of antimalarial drugs when visitors or returning indigenous people to West Africa or even resident indigenous people, use the drugs developed for the radical cure of acute malaria disease, as prophylactic, that is, taking the drug to prevent infection. Widespread prophylactic use of drugs can lead to the parasite becoming exposed to sub-clinical doses of the drug, and hence to the emergence of drug resistance. Plasmodium falciparum resistance to chloroquine is thought to have been triggered by the prophylactic use of the drug. Some countries, notably Brazil, attempted mass prophylaxis of their population by including it in table salt!

iii. Herbal remedies as antimalarial or adjunct to antimalarial drug therapy

We have speculated in this book that traditional African herbal treatment of malaria-induced fever, aches and pains (inflammation) was, in the traditional African setting, tantamount to cure of the disease in the partially immune person. There is evidence that tumour necrosis factor (TNF), one of the cytokines most extensively cited as a major pro-inflammatory agent in falciparum malaria can cause immuno-suppression in addition to the classic symptoms of malaria disease—fever and rigours, headache, myalgia, thrombo-cytopenia, etc. Following the amelioration of inflammation, the immune system of the partially immune person would surge and eliminate the parasite. Even though there is no direct empirical placebo controlled proof of this hypothesis, the historical fact that Africans in malaria endemic areas definitely survived on herbal treatment before the advent of modern chemotherapy gives the suggestion a strong plausibility. Even now, many Nigerians rely on herbal concoctions such as agbo or uhunvwun for the treatment of fever. Furthermore, the finding that commonly used traditional herbal remedies possess anti-inflammatory properties and, the pathology of malaria disease has been shown to be underpinned by inflammation mechanisms, is strong circumstantial evidence in support of the hypothesis which thus presents a challenge and an opportunity to the Nigerian community of medical scientists, the pharmaceutical industry and Nigerian governments to seriously undertake developmental programmes to carefully analyse the anti-inflammatory profiles of the anti-fever plant remedies known widely in Nigerian communities.

Let me stress that anti-fever herbal remedies are not being touted here as a panacea for all malaria disease sufferers. Even in sub-Saharan Africa there are subsets of the indigenous population in whom immunity may be compromised such as people in the extremes of age, pregnant women and people living with HIV/AIDS and tuberculosis that must always require special considerations. But for the benefit of a vast majority of adult Nigerians who possess partial immunity, a concerted effort to develop anti-inflammatory plant remedies would be a worthy effort. Nigerian scientists and governments would then be engaged in a development project whose concept has its origins in indigenous practice, and sound scientific premise and that has, among other advantages (see above), the potential to minimize resistance to expensive plasmodicidal drugs. Such herbal remedies if properly developed could be used solely as antimalarial therapy or as adjunct therapy to other conventional treatments.

Inflammation as an important component of the pathology of malaria and other diseases is a complex phenomenon; existing non-steroidal anti-inflammatory drugs (NSAIDs) such as ibuprofen and aspirin which act specifically on the cyclooxygenase pathway are therefore not the answer. Because plant remedies possess a cocktail of chemical constituents with a wide variety of anti-inflammatory mechanisms, natural products are now a major focus worldwide in the search for anti-inflammatories for the treatment of diseases in which inflammation mechanisms are a core component of pathology.

Afterword and Recommendations

I t is impossible to know with any certainty how African ancients arrived at beliefs, such as the Africa-wide belief that angered ancestors can punish an offending descendant with serious illness (ancestor spirit anger belief), and at other concepts pertaining to health and illness that are described in this book. But it can safely be assumed that those beliefs resulted from millennia of observation and experience of disease in the African environment and must, from an evolutionary and ecological perspective, be considered rational. That is to say, the beliefs evolved from ideas that most enabled the people to survive in their ecological niches. The core ideas which seem to satisfy these survival imperatives are embedded in the ancestor spirit anger belief, which I have interpreted as a metaphor for sustained emotional distress. This interpretation enables us to grasp the basic principles of traditional African medicine and its importance for health research in modern medicine for the benefit of the African people.

Africans have been conditioned into accepting the view that there is nothing of value in ancient African institutions, a view that came into being 500 years ago, in an environment of racial prejudice, bigotry and ignorance of the importance of these institutions. This negative view of Africa continues to be reinforced by the religious and education curricula left behind by former colonial rulers, and by Africa's continued total reliance, since independence, on Euro-American-dominated institutions for ideas on how to tackle Africa's problems. The ideas which guided life here for millennia before European contact are portrayed as superstitions in conflict with the major imported religious faiths and that cannot serve as models on which to build Africa's modern institutions. This mindset that Africa's ancient beliefs and institutions can have no relevance to today's problems ignores the importance of the physical environment and culture in the evolution of ideas. Unfortunately this mindset still persists among the African intelligentsia. In this book I have advanced arguments which debunk the assumption that African beliefs in relation to health are mindless superstitions.

The educated African elite who now guide 'development' on the continent, have internalized the negative view of Africa's past to a remarkable degree. We frequently behave as if we actually accept the view that the African mind was blank, devoid of any ideas, before Europe came to write its culture on it. Thus no serious thought is given to how Africans managed their affairs (in governance, medicine, agriculture, diplomacy, science, technology, etc) before Europeans came here. All our models of development, inappropriate as they often turn out to be, are Euro-American models. This is a tragedy because what we are talking about is the rejection of a peoples' culture by the people themselves. Culture has been defined as "the totality of socially transmitted behaviour patterns, art, beliefs, institutions, and all other products of human work and thought". In that sense culture defines a people as a historical entity. Therefore, a rejection of the accumulated African experience, of African culture as it had evolved before European contact by Africans themselves, is tantamount to a rejection of the self. It is like saying we did not exist before European intervention and are now attempting to recreate the African in a new European image. This remodelling attempt in which we are forced to portray ancient African beliefs, myths and esoteric practices as mindless superstitions, not worthy of serious contemplation, is largely responsible for Africa's failure in the world today.

The accumulated experiences and thoughts formulated as beliefs are rational products of an evolutionary process embodying ideas that are relevant to Africa's problems today. After all, we still live in Africa! This is the core proposition in this book. I argue that the evolution of culture as defined above is akin to the evolution of living organisms and obeys Darwinian principles; that is, the cultural elements (beliefs, thoughts and practices, etc) that survived evolutionary selection pressures, are those elements that enabled the African people to survive best in particular environments. This is the explanation for the cultural diversity that we observe among peoples of the world. The denial of the worth of the African past which began with European contact 500 years ago was thus a human tragedy of immeasurable proportion.

Malaria disease which is discussed extensively in this book is just one example of instances where the African elite have failed to draw on traditional African experience and knowledge in attempts to solve problems that face the African people. The scholar in the African university has the greatest opportunity as well as the responsibility and duty to address this deficiency, at the root of which is the education curriculum. A radical rethink of the curriculum is where the resolution of the African dilemma must start. The mind of the African child embarking on western education in colonial times was, and to some extent even now assumed, like the slate in his hand, to be blank, or if it happened that it was not blank, then it was to be wiped clean of its content of any indigenous knowledge by subtle mechanisms, so that it can be filled with European culture. We of the older generation are witnesses to the environment where vernacular (the native language) was prohibited in the school premises. Aspects of that curriculum still persists serving as a mechanism for the European cultural domination of the mind of the educated African elite.

The challenge for all of us now, especially the African scholar, is how to rework the curriculum radically so that African thought and philosophies developed over millennia in the environment of African culture, and crystallized as songs, myths, beliefs, fables, taboos can be engaged and explored, not just as intellectual exercise to generate publications, but as foundations for the new education aimed at liberating the African from the bondage of colonial indoctrination.

Recommendations

A book such as this, where the main aim has been to explore meanings in the symbols, beliefs, esoteric concepts and processes in traditional African medicine, is probably not the place for recommendations whose implementation may have policy implications. My doubts in this respect are due to the fact that these recommendations are based on inferences and claims of effectiveness of indigenous African therapeutic models that have not been empirically authenticated. On reflection however, I have included these two sets of recommendations for their importance to Africa's immediate and long-term health needs.

i. Establish a National Centre for Inflammation and Malaria Research (NCIMR)

I have speculated that over millennia indigenous African people acquired the knowledge, through experience, of the use of herbal remedies to treat fever, a quintessential manifestation of inflammation and a characteristic symptom of malaria disease. As matters have turned out, there is much evidence that malaria is an inflammatory disease; that is to say, its pathology is underpinned by inflammation mechanisms. Intuition also led African people to identify and use, in their various communities, plants which are now known to have anti-fever/anti-inflammatory properties. This is an important coincidence of African intuition and science, which should inspire individual scientists into action. However, malaria research is of such vital importance to Nigeria or it should be that it must be tackled with concerted effort at the national level using all available resources and from different perspectives. After all, when it is said, repeatedly, that the vast majority of all deaths due to malaria occur in sub-Saharan Africa, Nigeria as the epicenter of the disease, probably contributes 90% of those deaths, hence this recommendation: I am under no illusion that NCIMR will come into existence any time soon, but I am convinced that this book is where to set down the detailed rational basis for its recommendation.

The recent findings that

(i) inflammation is an important component of malaria pathology, and

(ii) that many of the plants used by local communities in Nigeria to treat malaria/fever possess anti-inflammatory properties, which I hypothesize, may account for the clinical effectiveness of such plants in the partially immune African, point to a new paradigm for malaria research; which is, to direct attention to the search for plants or a combination of plants that can be used, either in the crude form or as purified extracts, to effectively control malaria-induced inflammation. In conventional protocols where the search is for plasmodicidal chemical entities (substances that kill the plasmodium), plant extracts possessing demonstrable anti-inflammatory properties may be put aside as not interesting enough for further investigation. I am suggesting that the possession of anti-inflammatory properties should now be of utmost interest in the treatment of malaria disease in the partially immune African living in endemic areas.

But, to take full advantage of the new insight, we have to bear in mind two important points: The first is that inflammation is a complex biological phenomenon in which many different mechanisms play different parts. If we are to exploit the fortuitous abundance of known anti-fever/antimalarial plants in our communities as potential anti-inflammatory therapies or as adjunct to convential treatments, we need, deliberately, to build the capacity for research in inflammation science. This is in order to better understand which steps in the inflammation cascade are affected by the many groups of anti-inflammatory chemical entities which are known to be present in anti-fever plants. We know that plant extracts with anti-inflammatory properties act against many different inflammation mechanisms (see the review in this book by Peter Akah and Chukwuemeka, appendix 2 (pp.329-358). Also, we must understand the nature of the inflammation cascade in malaria disease itself. The whole problem calls for a deliberate establishment of a centre for inflammation research. The importance of such a centre does not lie in the understanding of malaria alone for, as indicated above, inflammation mechanisms also underlie the pathology of many other important diseases. This is an area of scientific endeavour in which potentially significant contributions to modern medicine can be made by Nigerian scientists.

In this book I have taken the liberty to speculate a great deal, admittedly not always on the basis of empirical evidence, that there are lessons that could be learnt if we examined the traditional African experience in the area of health. I have taken the view that some such speculation must be permissible in attempting to interpret ancient practices that were based on oral tradition and expressed in religious beliefs in forms that were designed essentially more for mnemonic rather than clarity purposes. My view is that the speculations should be examined for consistency and where possible, tested in basic pre-clinical and clinical experimental protocols. That seems to me to be a valid way to proceed to discover the useful lessons to be learnt from the accumulated African experience in the area of health.

One such speculation is that the traditional African herbal treatment of malaria/fever was an appropriate therapeutic approach for people living in malaria endemic environments. It merits further study and possible verification because it is a treatment strategy that avoided provoking the plasmodium parasite into mobilizing its considerable innate resistance mechanisms, and because it ensured the continuous maintenance of the partial immunity of individuals in that environment. If this was shown empirically to be valid, it would explain how Africans in malaria endemic areas survived and lived in equilibrium with malaria disease before the advent of modern chemotherapy. An attempt at validation of the hypothesis provides an opportunity to focus research on the phenomenon of inflammation which underpins the pathology of malaria. It is also an opportunity to test the much touted curative power of traditional herbal treatments, in properly conducted clinical trials in a way that has not been done before. It is on this basis that the case for the establishment of an institute or centre dedicated to the study and research into malaria disease and inflammation is made. Such an institute would tackle malaria research from an indigenous experience perspective and more likely to receive international attention than our copycat approaches so far.

There is also a wider issue: It has always been assumed that plants used in traditional medicine in Africa should yield drugs for the treatment of different diseases. This expectation is based on the premise that if the plants worked in their crude forms in traditional usage, they must contain drug-like chemical entities, and given modern technology with which to extract the active ingredients, production of drugs from such plants should be a straightforward matter such that Africa with so many forests should be self sufficient in the area of drugs. This thinking has lured many scientists and institutions worldwide into developing protocols and devoting huge resources for the search for drugs in African medicinal plants.

In the past 4 or 5 decades during which this thinking has dominated research in traditional medicine in Africa, there have been many interesting scientific publications, many exaggerated claims, but no drugs of any real importance have been discovered. Many reasons can be given for this failure— insufficient funding, inadequate expertise etc. But there is also a fundamental issue: In using herbal remedies in TAM and drugs in modern medicine respectively, two different treatment objectives are in operation, particularly in the treatment of chronic life-threatening illness whose cause, in the case of traditional African medicine, cannot be determined with certainty. In modern medicine, the drug is used in such circumstances to remove the identified cause of disease by selectively poisoning it, whereas the herbal remedy in the treatment of serious illness in TAM is best understood as a part of the treatment assemblage which includes esoteric practices meant to diffuse emotional distress. Thus if we want to be guided by traditional practice in our search for e.g. antimalarial drugs in plants, we should not be looking for plant extracts that kill the plasmodium (it would be fortunate if we did discover such chemical entities!); but such plants would most likely be poisonous and would have been omitted from the traditional pharmacopeia of plant remedies (see p...) and not used by traditional healers to treat malaria. We should be searching for chemical entities that cure the symptoms of malaria infection. We should reason that if the plant extract is effective against fever, it almost certainly contains an anti-inflammatory motif (fever is the quintessential expression of inflammation). In the last 3 decades or so Nigerian scientists have shown, in simple animal models, that extracts of plants used in the treatment of fever (including, obviously, malaria fever) do possess anti-inflammatory properties (see appendix 2, pages 329-358).

The core of my argument in recommending the establishment of a centre for malaria and inflammation research is this: Treating the underlying inflammation component of malaria disease is an approach to malaria therapy that has its origins in African indigenous experience, with the likelihood that in the partially immune adult African person, such treatment amounted to cure. Although this suggestion has not been directly proven, it is a plausible working hypothesis. What is more, inflammation now appears to be a major component of the pathology, not only of malaria, one of Africa's oldest and most important maladies, but also of many other diseases known to modern medicine. And, we have an abundance of plants in Nigerian communities that seem, from preliminary research, to possess anti-inflammatory properties. Thus inflammation is one field of medical research in which Nigeria can invest with the real possibility of both economic and intellectual returns. What is needed therefore is a capability, preferably a purpose-built institute or centre, to enable scientists to have access to the necessary technology to undertake in-depth research into the nature of inflammation and to test the hypothesis in preclinical laboratory and clinical studies. Inflammation is an important emerging discipline in medical science with particular relevance to important diseases that are prevalent in this environment. Therefore, Nigerian medical scientists should be empowered to take active part in it.

A fair counter argument can be made that there are two health related research institutes in Nigeria which can take care of the problems to be tackled by the proposed NCIMR: The Nigerian Institute for Pharmaceutical Research & Drug Production (NIPRD) and the Nigerian Institute for Medical Research (NIMR) originally West African Council for Medical Research (WCMR). My view is that these two research institutes have broader objectives. Their existence should not preclude the establishment of the NCIMR whose objective is narrower and specifically focused on the phenomenon of inflammation and malaria disease, and should complement NIPRD and NIMR.

ii. Inclusion of basic principles of traditional African
medicine in the curricula for the training of health
personnel in colleges of medicine and pharmacy

The cultures of medicine have evolved among different human populations throughout history. The ideas pertaining to illness that survived the passage of time were those that the people found to be most beneficial in the treatment of the diseases that were most frequently experienced by the people in their different environments. Therefore, from the point of view of ecological and cultural relevance, traditional African medicine ought to have been the foundation on which modern medicine in Africa is grounded. Unfortunately, not only is this not the case, to make matters more tragic, traditional African medicine is actually denigrated by African modern men and women.

At the point of contact with modern medicine in Africa, the peoples' ideas on illness were dismissed as superstition, not worthy of inclusion in syllabuses designed for the training of modern African medical personnel. The African elite, particularly those trained in the principles of modern medicine, generally acquiesced in the European denigration of traditional African thoughts on illness as nothing more than expressions of ignorance. Consequently, after more than five decades of independence from colonial bondage—enough time for us to have recovered from colonial indoctrination into a consciousness of our cultural heritage in matters of African thoughts on causes of illness—no reference is made to traditional African medicine in African colleges of medicine and pharmacy. One would have thought that by now, these syllabuses should, at the very least, acknowledge the existence of TAM's huge body of knowledge, whether we understand it all or not. The omission of TAM from our curricula is a tragic flaw for several reasons.

First, as discussed extensively in the body of this book, the ancestor spirit anger belief, for example, is a crystallization of the idea that links life-threatening illness to sustained emotional distress in traditional African thought. Sustained emotional distress is also now recognized as a risk factor for the occurrence of chronic diseases such as cancer and cardiovascular and metabolic diseases in modern medicine. Now, emotional distress is a condition that typically arises from strains in interpersonal relationships. A recognition of this principle in traditional African thought since ancient times, suggests that proneness to emotional distress may well be of particular importance as a risk factor among African populations, who have historically struggled to cope with culture conflicts and dramatically changing lifestyles. Now, even more than ever before, African populations endure emotional and physical stresses in their daily lives. The new modern medicine discipline of psychoneuroimmunology (or brain control of host immunity) which is using modern tools to map out the pathways that link emotions to a person's physical state of health should feature in the curriculum of African colleges of medicine and pharmacy. At an appropriate level of training, the subject of emotion and health should be introduced in the syllabus; a good starting point would be a discussion of the Africa-wide belief in

ancestor spirit anger as an explanation for the occurrence
of chronic illness and the interpretation of the belief
presented here can serve as a platform on which the
science of psychoneuroimmunology can be based.

The other reason why the basic principles of TAM
should feature in the training curricula of health
personnel in Africa is the fact that the ideas embedded in
African beliefs regarding health, as described in this
book, are interesting from an ecological/evolutionary
standpoint and are therefore worthy of further
exploration. Exposing young imaginations to those ideas
is the surest way to keep them alive in the context of
advances in modern medicine.

Furthermore, it would be beneficial to both the health
practitioner and the patient in Africa if the former is
exposed to TAM ideas during the training period. Such
exposure would provide him/her with the opportunity to
compare the two systems. And, the practitioner would be
better at dealing with patients, many of whom come from
a background in which they have had considerable
exposure to TAM and traditional African ideas about
illness and its treatment. As I have pointed out in the
book, ideas and habits internalized from TAM can
interact with modern medicine in complex ways,
sometimes, with disastrous consequences.

Introduction to Chukwuemeka Sylvestor Nworu and Peter Achunike Akah's Review

The inflammation reaction is a complex biological phenomenon that is usually described simply as the response of a living cell to injury. Medical interest in inflammation arises from the fact that the pharmacological activities of the mediators of inflammation often manifest as disease requiring therapeutic intervention.

Inflammation is a complex subject because different types of living cells experience different types of injury in their interactions with various elements in the external and internal melieu, and each cell type responds with a mechanism appropriate to its situation.

In man at least, inflammation seems to function as a defence mechanism, as an evolutionary survival device, e.g, to remove the cause of injury (bacteria, virus, antigen-antibody complex, etc), to prevent the spread of the injury, or to draw attention to the injury so that the sufferer may do something to prevent further damage (fever, aches and pains). Because the living cells in different organs of the body must experience different types of injury frequently and inflammation is the initial response in every case, it is not surprising that inflammation is a major component of the pathology of many human diseases. It is important to emphasize that the inflammatory mechanisms in one disease may differ from those in another; thus, although diseases may be classed together as inflammatory diseases because their pathologies are underpinned by inflammatory mechanisms, different classes of anti-inflammatory drugs may be required to treat each disease in the class because of the differences in underlying mechanisms: for example, as has been pointed out already, although asthma and rheumatoid arthritis are described as inflammatory diseases, the detailed inflammation mechanisms are different and the anti-inflammatory drugs for their treatment belong to different classes (steroidal antiinflammatories for asthma and NSAIDs for rheumatoid arthritis). In fact, NSAIDs may make asthma worse.

Academic university departments and drug discovery outfits in the pharmaceutical industry are trying to develop drugs that block specific inflammation mechanistic pathways for use in the treatment of inflammatory diseases; but it is very unlikely that we shall soon have an anti-inflammatory equivalent of the 'magic bullet' for the treatment of all the diseases in which inflammation plays a key role. The search for such a drug would be like the search for the holy grail of medicine. This is why science is turning to the plant kingdom as a source of anti-inflammatories. Chukuemeka Nworu and Peter Akah's contribution that follows is a review of the extraordinary array of inflammation mechanisms that can be inhibited by chemical entities present in plants.

If inflammation by definition, is the response of the living cell to injury, it is understandable that inflammation contributes to the pathologies of virtually all chronic diseases in the aging organism. This is implicit in Selye's description of illness as a non-specific adaptation syndrome, an attempt by the human body to fight an infection or injury. Illness is not due to the infection per se but the body's response to it, to put up a fight against the injury, without the body's fight, there would be no illness. Inflammation, in other words, is the mechanism used by the body to contain infection. Recent evidence suggests that many debilitating diseases can be classed as inflammatory diseases, including many cancers, Parkinson's disease, malaria, sickle cell disease, Alzheimer's disease etc., because the pathologies in these diseases are underpinned by inflammation mechanisms.

The reason why science is turning attention to the plant kingdom in the search for anti-inflammatory entities is that plants, like humans, must endure cellular injuries of the type that provoke inflammation. Plants have, therefore, over evolutionary time developed the capacity to make anti-inflammatory chemical entities which they store as protection against injury. It is not a surprise that anti-inflammatories with an outstandingly broad range of activities abound in the plant kingdom.

Appendix 2
Anti-inflammatory Herbs and Their Molecular Mechanisms of Action

Chukwuemeka Sylvester Nworu & Peter Achunike Akah

Department of Pharmacology & Toxicology,
Faculty of Pharmaceutical Sciences,
University of Nigeria, Nsukka

ABSTRACT

A large number of studies have shown that anti-inflammatory activities of herbal extracts and herb-derived compounds are mainly due to their inhibition of arachidonic acid (AA) metabolism, cyclo-oxygenase (COX), lipo-oxygenase (LOX), pro-inflammatory cytokines, inducible nitric oxide, and transcription activation factor (NF-κB). Some anti-inflammatory medicinal herbs are reported to stabilize lysosomal membrane and some cause the uncoupling of oxidative phosphorylation of intracellular signalling molecules. Many have also been shown to possess strong oxygen radical scavenging activities. Most of these mechanisms are related and many herbal products have been shown to act through a combination of these molecular pathways. Interestingly, many of these herbs lack the gastro-erosive side effects of non-steroidal anti-inflammatory drugs (NSAID) or the plethora of unwanted side effects associated with steroidal anti-inflammatory drugs. For these reasons, medicinal plant and plant products have shown tremendous potentials and are used beneficially in the treatment of

inflammation and in the management of diseases with
significant inflammatory components. This chapter is to
review some anti-inflammatory herbs and their molecular
mechanisms of action.

Introduction

There are several proposed cellular mechanisms explaining in
vivo anti-inflammatory activity of medicinal plants. These
mechanisms include antioxidative and radical scavenging
activities, regulation of cellular activities of the inflammation-
related cells: mast cells, macrophages, lymphocytes, and
neutrophils (for instance, some inhibit histamine release from
mast cells and others inhibit T-cell proliferation), modulation
of the enzymatic activities of arachidonic acid (AA)
metabolizing enzymes such as phospholipase A2 (PLA2),
cyclooxygenase (COX), and lipoxygenase (LOX) and the nitric
oxide (NO) producing enzyme, nitric oxide synthase (NOS)
(Vane and Botting, 1987; Chen, 2011). The inhibition of these
enzymes by anti-inflammatory medicinal plant products
(AIMP) reduce the production of AA, prostaglandins (PG),
leukotrienes (LT), and NO, which are crucial mediators of
inflammation (Khanapure et al, 2007). Thus, the inhibition of
these enzymes by AIMP is one of the important cellular
mechanisms of anti-inflammation. In recent years, many lines
of evidence support the idea that certain AIMP are the
modulators of gene expression, especially the modulators of
pro-inflammatory gene expression, thus leading to the
attenuation of the inflammatory response. Here, we have
highlighted the relevance of these mechanisms as they are
related to the activities of herbal products used in the
treatment of inflammation.

1.0 Inhibition of Phospholipase A2

During an inflammatory response, arachidonic acid (AA), a precursor of eicosanoids, is released mostly from membrane lipids in cells. The enzyme responsible for this release is Phospholipase A2 (PLA2), although some portion is attributed to the combined action of phospholipase C and diacylglycerol lipase (Ito et al, 2002). AA mobilization by PLA2 and subsequent prostaglandins' synthesis is considered to be a pivotal event in inflammation. Therefore, drugs that inhibit PLA2 thus block the cyclo-oxygenase (COX) and lipo-oxygenase (LOX) pathways in the AA cascade are effective in the treatment of inflammatory processes. PLA2 catalyses the hydrolysis of the acyl group attached to the 2-position of intracellular membrane phosphoglycerides which releases arachidonic acid from membrane phosphoglycerides. Arachidonic acid is the precursor of prostaglandins (PGs), thromboxanes, and leukotrienes. Some anti-inflammatory medicinal plants inhibit PLA2 (figure 1) and this inhibition is mediated via lipocortin or by direct interaction with the enzyme itself. The former mechanism utilizes a protein known as lipocortin, the synthesis of which is induced by steroidal hormones and steroidal plant metabolite, triterpenoids (Barnes, 1998). The other mechanism involves a direct binding with the enzyme itself, a mechanism that is yet to be exploited in therapeutics but with great promise. It is known that betulinic acid, a triterpene act by direct binding to phospholipase A2 (Wiart, 2006).

The inhibitory activity of several flavonoid derivatives against AA metabolizing enzymes was initially reported in 1980 (Bauman et al, 1980). Thereafter, investigators have studied the inhibitory effect of flavonoids on these enzymes (Kim et al, 2004). Up to date, many isoforms of PLA2 have been discovered (Murakami and Kudo, 2004). They are mainly classified into three large categories, secretory PLA2 (sPLA2), cytosolic PLA2 (cPLA2), and calcium independent PLA2 (iPLA2). These PLA2s are distributed in wide varieties of tissues and cells. In some conditions, they are coupled to COXs depending on the cells and agonists used (Murakami and Kudo, 2004). For instance, group IIA sPLA2 was found in arthritic synovial fluid, and group IV cPLA2 are coupled to COXs and 5-LOX to produce eicosanoids (Murakami and Kudo, 2004). Therefore, a modulation of sPLA2 and/or cPLA2 activity is important in the control of inflammatory processes.

The first flavonoid inhibitor of PLA2 to be identified was quercetin, which inhibited PLA2 from human neutrophils (Lee et al, 1982). Quercetin was repeatedly found to inhibit PLA2 from several sources. It inhibited PLA2 from rabbit peritoneal neutrophils with an IC50 of 57-100 μM (Lanni and Becker, 1985). It was also demonstrated that quercetin selectively inhibited group II sPLA2 from Vipera russelli with less inhibition of PLA2 from porcine pancreas, PLA2-IB (Lindahl and Tagesson, 1993). While flavanones including flavanone, hesperetin, and naringenin showed less inhibition, flavonols such as kaempferol, quercetin, and myricetin were found to considerably inhibit snake venom PLA2, indicating an importance of the C-ring-2,3-double bond (Welton et al, 1986).

In many other studies, other herbal extracts and phytocontituents have been reported to exhibit significant anti-inflammatory effects through an inhibition of various PLA2. Extract of Trichilia catigua (Meliaceae) completely inhibited PLA2 at a concentration of 120 μg/ml (Barbosa et al, 2004). Ethanol extract of Baccharis uncinella DC (Asteraceae) were reported to contain among other constituents two triterpenoids (oleanolic and ursolic acids) and one flavonoid (pectolinaringenin) which exhibited anti-inflammatory effects against inflammatory reactions induced by phospholipase A2 (from Crotalus durissus terrificus venom) (Zalewski et al, 2011). It was shown recently that the water extract of Aloe vera leaf skin (AVLS) extract exhibited anti- PLA2 activity with an

IC50 = 0.22 mg/ml (Kammoun et al, 2011). Also recently, it was shown that the neuroprotective effect of Ginkgo biloba extract (EGb761) was mediated, at least in part, through inhibition of cytosolic cPLA2 activation (Zhao et al, 2011). In a study to evaluate the effects of the flavonoid, quercetin, on Crotalus durissus terrificus secretory phospholipase A2 (sPLA2), it was reported that the protein was chemically modified by treatment with quercetin, which resulted in modifications in the secondary structure as evidenced through circular dichroism (Kim et al, 2004). In addition, quercetin was able to inhibit the enzymatic activity and some pharmacological activities of sPLA2, including its antibacterial activity, its ability to induce platelet aggregation, and its myotoxicity by approximately 40% (Cotrim et al, 2011). Cochinchina momordica seed extract (SKMS10) was also shown to exhibit anti-inflammatory activities by down-regulating cPLA2 among other molecular mechanisms of action (Kang et al, 2009).

2.0 Inhibitors of cyclooxygenases (COX)

COX that produces prosaglandins (PGs) and thromboxanes (TX) from arachidonic acid exists in two different isoforms (COX-1 and -2). COX-1 is a constitutive enzyme existing in almost every cell type, catalysing the conversion of AA into cytoprotective PGs and blood pro-aggregatory TXs. On the other hand, COX-2 is an inducible enzyme and in most cases causes the production of a large amount of PGs (Needleman and Isakson, 1997). COX-2 is highly expressed in the inflammation-related cell types including macrophages and mast cells, when they are stimulated with pro-inflammatory cytokines and/or bacterial lipopolysaccharide (LPS) (Needleman and Isakson, 1997). The inhibition of both COX-1 and COX-2 has been found to be the molecular target of many anti-inflammatory herbal extracts and herb-derived compounds (figure 1). COX-2 that produces PGs is closely associated with inflammatory disorders of acute as well as chronic types. Actually, COX-2 selective inhibitors possess anti-inflammatory activity with reduced side effects frequently seen with COX-1/COX-2 non-selective inhibitors (McMurray and Hardy, 2002).

Devil's claw, Harpagophytum procumbens DC (Pedaliaceae), used in South Africa for the management of pain and inflammation, is an example of medicinal plant whose anti-inflammatory activities is based on reported inhibition of COX (Kundu et al, 2005). Anti-inflammatory effects of seven lignans and one dihydrochalcone isolated from the leaves of two Lauraceae species (Pleurothyrium cinereum and Ocotea macrophylla), were found to be potent inhibitors of COX-2/5-LOX (Coy-Barrera and Cuca-Suarez, 2011). Ethyl acetate-soluble extract of the stems of Macrococculus pomiferus was found to inhibit COX-2 (Su et al, 2004). (S)-coriolic acid and

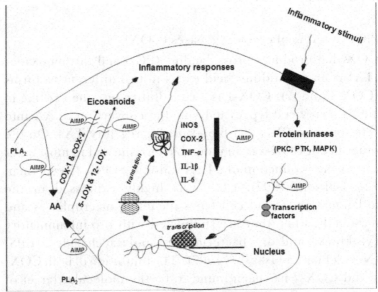

Figure 1. The proposed mechanism of action of anti-inflammatory medicinal plants (AIMP). "≈ " and " ↓ " denote enzyme inhibition and down-regulation of the expression, respe

(+/-)-glycerol 1-monolinolate isolated from ethylacetate-soluble extract of the seeds of Hernandia ovigera showed selective inhibitory activity with cyclooxygenase-2 (Jang et al, 2004). The compound, 2, 4, 5-trimethoxybenzaldehyde, isolated from Daucus carota seed extracts, inhibited COX-2 enzyme very significantly at a concentration of 100 µg/ml (Momin et al, 2003). Some flavonoids such as luteolin, 3', 4'-dihyroxyflavone, galangin, and morin were found as inhibitors of COX (Bauman et al, 1980). When their structural activity relationships were compared, several flavone derivatives such as flavone and apigenin were found to be COX inhibitors, while some flavonol derivatives such as quercetin and myricetin were preferential LOX inhibitors. Also, certain flavonoids such as flavone, kaempferol, and quercetin were repeatedly found to be inhibitors of COX from rat peritoneal macrophages (Welton et al, 1986). After these reports, many studies have been done to figure out the inhibitory activity of flavonoids on COX, mostly COX-1. For instance, flavonoids such as quercetin and xanthomicrol were reported to inhibit sheep platelet COX-1; while the IC50 values of flavones such as cirsiliol, hypolaetin, and diosmetin were more than 100 µM (Ferrandiz et al, 1990). Furthermore, flavones and flavonols including chrysin, flavone, galangin, kaempferol, and quercetin were repeatedly revealed to inhibit TXB2 formation from mixed leukocyte suspension probably by COX-1 inhibition (Laughton et al, 1991).

3.0 Inhibition of lipoxygenases (LOX)

Arachidonate 5-lipoxygenase is the key enzyme in leukotriene biosynthesis and catalyses the initial steps in the conversion of arachidonic acid to biologically active leukotrienes. Leukotrienes are considered as potent mediators of inflammatory and allergic reactions, and regarding their pro-inflammatory properties the inhibition of 5-lipoxygenase pathway is considered to be interesting in the treatment of a variety of inflammatory diseases. Lipoxygenases (LOX) are present in leucocytes, tracheal cells, keratinocytes, and the epithelium of stomach and airways and they catalyse the introduction of a molecule of oxygen to the 5-position of AA to give the intermediate 5(S)- hydroxy-(6E, 8Z, 11Z, 14Z)-eicosatetraenoic acid, 5-HETE, which is immediately followed by the re-arrangement of 5-HETE to leukotrienes. This is another target for anti-inflammatory medicinal plants that inhibit the biogenesis of leukotrienes and 5-HETE (figure 1). Medicinal plants that inhibit LOX hold some other useful therapeutic potential in the treatment of asthma, psoriasis, arthritis, allergic rhinitis, cancer, osteoporosis, and artherosclerosis.

A potential source for new 5-lipoxygenase inhibitors is undoubtedly provided by medicinal plants used in traditional medicine. The Arisia species and other Myrsinacea family produce very unusual series of dimeric benzoquinones known as ardisiaquinones, which are known to inhibit the enzymatic activity of 5-LOX. This feature could explain the frequent use of Ardisia species to treat inflammatory conditions. One such compound is Ardisiaquinone G which was isolated from Ardisia teysmanniana and is known to inhibit LOX (Yang et al, 2001; Fuuishi et al, 2001). The Asteraceae family is one of the richest sources of LOX inhibitors and three different types of principles exhibiting remarkable LOX inhibition have been isolated and characterized. Helenalin, a sesquiterpene lactone, which can be isolated from several plant species of the Asteraceae family possess potent anti-inflammatory and antineoplastic agent. Helenalin inhibited 5-LOX (IC_{50} 9 mM after a 60 minute preincubation) in a concentration and time-dependent fashion in human granulocyte culture (Tornhamre et al, 2001). Polyacetylenes from Artemisia monosperma showed some levels of activity against LOX (Stavri et al, 2005). The third group of LOX inhibitors in this family includes the bornyl cinnamoyl derivatives from Verbenisa species, such as bornyl caffeate from the South American herb Verbenisa turbacensis Kunth. Another compound, friedelin, isolated from the bark of Commiphora berryi, showed significant soybean lipoxygenase (SBL) inhibitory activity with IC 50 of $35.8\mu M$ (Kumari et al, 2011).

Generally, an enormous number of different plant-derived compounds from various species have been found to interfere with 5-LOX activities. In general, it appears that lipophylic, often fatty acid-like compounds with (i.e. phenols) and without (i.e. triterpenes and polyacetylenes) reducing properties interfere with 5-LOX and the majority are phenolic structures including flavonoids, quinones, (that become hydroxylated to hydroquinones), hydroxylated coumarines, and many other polyphenols. Apparently a combination of iron-reducing and iron-chelating properties of these phenolic compounds is responsible for 5-LOX inhibitions (Werz, 2007).

Table 1. Examples of some anti-inflammatory medicinal plants reported to inhibit 5-lipoxygenase.

Plant species/Family	Extract/plant part used	Active constituent/ fraction	References
Longifolia Nees (Asteracantha)	Methanol seed extract		Kumar et al, 2000
Gomphrena perennis L. (Amaranthaceae)	Methanol extract of aerial part	Ethylacetate fraction	Matsunaga et al, 2000
Vitis amurensis Rupr. (Ampelidaceae)	Ethanol root extract	Amurensin	Huang et al, 2000
Pistacia terebinthus L. (Anacardiaceae)	Methanol extract of gall	Masticadienolic acid, Morolic acid, Oleanolic acid	Giner-Larza et al, 2001; Giner-Larza et al, 2002
Toxicodendron radicans L. (Anacardiaceae)	Ethanol fruit extract	Urushiol	Wagner et al, 1989
Xylopia frutescens Aubl (Annonaceae)	n-Hexane seed extract		Braga et al, 2000
Ilex aquifolium L.	Ethanol leaf		Müller et al,

(Aquifoliaceae)	extract		1998
Achillea ageratifolia Boiss. (Asteraceae)		Hexadeca-2E,7Z-diene-10-ynoic acid Pyrrolide	Müller-Jakic et al, 1994
Echinacea purpurea (L.) Moench (Asteraceae)	Root	Polyunsaturated isobutylamides	Wagner et al, 1989
Cannabis sativa L (Cannabinaceae)		Cannipren	El Sohly et al, 1990
Phyllanthus emblica (Euphorbiaceae)	Diethyl ether leaf extract		Ihantola-Vormisto et al, 1997
Cassia fistula L. (Fabaceae)	Methanol fruit extract		Sunil Kumar and Müller, 1998
Salvia aethiopis L. (Lamiaceae)	Root	Aethiopinone	Benrezzouk et al, 2001
Allium cepa L. (Liliaceae)	Chloroform extract of the bulb	Methyl-1-propenylthiosulfinate, Propyl-1-propenylthiosulfinate, Cepaenes	Wagner et al, 1990
Allium sativum L. (Liliaceae)	Chloroform extract of the bulb	Methylajoene, Dimethylajoene, Ajoeene, Allicin	Sendl et al, 1992
Ardisia japonica Blume (Myrsinaceae)	Methanol extract of the wood	Ardisianone A and B, Maesanin	Fukuyama et al, 1993
Punica granatum L. (Punicaceae)	Seed oil	Flavonoids	Schubert et al, 1999
Solanum xanthocarpum Schrad. (Solanaceae)	Methanol leaf extract		Kumar et al, 2000
Curcuma longa L. (Zingiberaceae)	Petroleum ether extract of the rhizome	Curcumine	Ammon et al, 1992

4.0 Inhibition of nitric oxide synthetase (NOS)

The NOS is an important enzyme involved in the regulation of inflammation, vascular tone, neurotransmission, and cancer. NO is a toxic free radical that can cause substantial tissue damage in high concentration. In stroke, large amount of NO is released from nerve cells and causes extensive damage to surrounding tissues including neurones and myocytes (Shah et al, 2011).

The NO is biochemically generated via oxidation of the terminal guanidine nitrogen atom from L-arginine by NOS. NO is one of the cellular mediators of physiological and pathological process (Moncada et al, 1991; Nathan, 1992; Mollace et al, 2005). Three different isoforms of NOS are now recognized: endothelial NOS (eNOS), neuronal NOS (nNOS), and inducible NOS (iNOS) (Venema et al, 1997; Stuehr, 1999). The former two are constitutively expressed in the body, whereas the latter type is an inducible enzyme highly expressed by inflammatory stimuli in certain cells such as macrophages. iNOS is involved in overproduction of NO in response to pro-inflammatory mediators such as interleukine-1β (IL-1β), tumour necrosis factor-α (TNF-α), and bacterial lipopolysaccharide (LPS). While a small amount of NO synthesized by eNOS and nNOS is essential for maintaining normal body function (homeostasis), a significantly increased amount of NO synthesized by iNOS participates in provoking inflammatory process and acts synergistically with other inflammatory mediators (Mollace et al, 2005). Many herbal extracts and compounds of herbal origin have shown strong inhibition of iNOS and NO over-production (figure 1). Search for herb-based compounds which can reduce NO production by inhibiting iNOS without affecting eNOS or nNOS is very desirable for anti-inflammatory agents.

Recently, we reported the inhibition of inducible NO production by the methanol extract of Spondias mombin (Nworu et al, 2011). LPS-stimulated NO production by bone marrow-derived macrophages was significantly inhibited at 25 μg/ml and 100 μg/ml of the methanol extract (Nworu et al, 2011). Artemisinin, a sequiterpene used in the treatment of malaria was demonstrated to inhibit NO synthesis in cytokine-stimulated human astrocytoma T67 cells (Aldieri et al, 2003).

Several studies suggest that sequiterpene lactones inhibit NO synthetase. For example, ambrosanolides-type sequiterpene known as cumanin isolated from Ambrosia psilostachya inhibited NO activity with an IC_{50} value of 9.38 μM (Lastra et al, 2004). Ursolic acid and 2-α- hydroxy ursolic acid, triterpenes from Prunella vulgaris L., inhibited NO from murine leukaemic monocytes macrophages (RAW 264.7) with IC_{50} of 17 μM and 27 μM, respectively (Ryu et al, 2000). Bigelovin, 2,3-dihydroaromaticin, and ergolide isolated from Inula species showed potent inhibition of LPS-induced NOS in RAW 264.7 cells with IC_{50} values of 0.46 mM, 1.05 mM, and 0.69 mM, respectively (Lee et al, 2002).

Inhibition of iNOS is not a general behaviour of flavonoids, but they inhibit NO production which means they down-regulate the expression of iNOS and not the activity of already produced enzymes. Flavone and several other amino-substituted flavones were reported to inhibit NO production (Krol et al, 1995). Flavonoids that down-regulate iNOS expression include flavones such as apigenin and oroxylin A; flavonols such as kaempferol and quercetin; biflavonoids such as bilobetin and ginkgetin, and some prenylated flavonoid such as sanggenons and kuwanon C (Kim et al, 2004).

5.0 Inhibitions of pro-inflammatory cytokines

A number of cytokines are associated with inflammatory diseases. Some pro-inflammatory cytokines also regulate inflammatory reactions either directly or by their ability to induce the synthesis of cellular adhesion molecules or other cytokines in certain cell types. The major pro-inflammatory cytokines that are responsible for early responses are IL1-alpha (IL-1α), IL1-beta (IL-1 β), IL-6, and TNF-alpha (TNF-α). Other pro-inflammatory mediators include leukemia inhibitory factor, (LIF), interferon-gamma (IFN-γ), oncostatin M (OSM), ciliary neurotrophic factor (CNTF), tumour growth factor-beta (TGF-β), granulocyte macrophage colony-stimulating factor (GM-CSF), IL-8, IL-11, IL-12, IL-17, IL-18, and a variety of other chemokines that chemoattractant inflammatory cells. Inhibition of the expression of these cytokines has been demonstrated as the target for many anti-inflammatory medicinal plants and their compounds (figure 1, table 1). Steroidal anti-inflammatory drugs (SAIDs) such as prednisolone and dexamethasone are also known to reduce the production of these pro-inflammatory cytokines (Newton, 2000).

Table 2. Examples of some anti-inflammatory medicinal plants reported to decrease the expression of some pro-inflammatory cytokines

Cytokine	Medicinal plant	Model used	References
IL-1	Curcuma longa Polygala tenuifolia Smilax glabra Uncaria tomentosa	In vitro, Human In vitro, Murine Ex vivo, Human In vitro, Murine	Chan, 1995 Kim et al, 998 Jiang and Xu, 2003 Lemaire et al, 1999
IL-1α	Allium sativum	In vitro, Human	Hodge et al, 2002
IL-1β	Ampelopsis brevipedunculata Harpagophytum procumbens Ludwigia octovalvis Pinus maritima Rhus semialata Tabernaemontana divaricata	In vitro, Human In vitro, Human In vitro, Human In vitro, Murine In vitro, Human In vitro, Human	Kuo et al, 1999 Fiebich et al, 2001 Kuo et al, 1999 Cho et al, 2001 Kuo et al, 1999 Kuo et al, 1999
IL-6	Allium sativum	In vitro,	Hodge et al, 2002

	Plant	Model	Reference
	Astragalus membranaceus	Human	Shon et al, 2002
	Coptis spp.	In vitro, Human	Iizuka et al, 2000
	Harpagophytum procumbens	Human	Fiebich et al, 2001
		In vivo, Murine	
		In vitro, Human	
TNF	Acanthopanax senticosus	In vitro, Murine	Yi et al, 2002
	Acer nikoense	In vitro, Murine	Fujiki et al, 2003
	Allium sativum	In vitro, Human	Hodge et al, 2002
	Ampelopsis	In vitro, Human	Kuo et al, 1999
	Curcuma longa	In vitro, Human	Chan, 1995
	Dichroa febrifuga	In vitro, Murine	Kim et al, 2000
	Harpagophytum procumbens	In vitro, Human	Fiebich et al, 2001
	Ludwigia octovalvis	In vitro, Human	Kuo et al, 1999
	Perilla frutescens	In vivo, Murine	Ueda and Yamazaki, 1997
	Polygala tenuifolia	In vitro, Murine	Hong et al, 2002
	Polygala tenuifolia	In vitro, Human	Kim et al, 1998
	Rhus semialata	In vitro, Murine	Kuo et al, 1999
	Rosa davurica	In vitro, Murine	Kim et al, 1999
	Scutellaria baicalensis	In vivo, Murine	Kim et al, 2001
	Sinomenium acutum	In vitro, Murine	Kim et al, 1999
	Smilax glabra	In vitro, Murine	Jiang and Xu, 2003
	Tabernaemontana divaricata	In vitro, Human	Kuo et al, 1999
	Tinospora cordifolia	In vitro, Murine	Dhuley, 1997
	Uncaria tomentosa	In vitro, Murine	Sandoval et al, 2002
	Withania somnifera	In vitro, Murine	Davis and Kuttan, 999
		In vivo, Murine	
		In vitro, Murine	

		In vivo, Murine In vitro, Murine In vivo, Murine	
IL-8	Coriolus versicolor Curcuma longa (Curcumin) Paeonia suffruticosa	In vitro, Human In vitro, Human In vitro, Bovine	Hsieh et al, 2002 Hidaka et al, 2002 Oh et al, 2003
IL-12	Allium sativum	In vitro, Human	Hodge et al, 2002

6.0 Modulation of pro-inflammatory gene expression

The cellular mechanisms through which anti-inflammatory medicinal plants modulate gene expression have also been extensively studied. The most prominent points of cellular regulation affected by these herbs and herb-based compounds are the various protein kinases involved in signal transduction including protein kinase C (PKC) and mitogen activated protein kinase (MAPK) (figure 1). Through the inhibition of these enzymes, DNA-binding capacity of transcription factors such as nuclear factor-B (NF-B) or activator protein-1 (AP-1) is regulated (Kim et al, 2004). Thereby, the expression rate of the target gene is controlled. Flavonoids inhibit the enzyme activities of various signal transduction protein kinases (Kim et al, 2004). The best example is PKC inhibition (Ferriola et al, 1989) and protein tyrosine kinase inhibition (Chang and Geahlen, 1992) by various flavonoid derivatives. MAPKs are also key elements in signal transduction. In macrophages, LPS activates three kinds of MAPKs, extracellular signal related kinase (ERK), p38 MAPK, and Jun N-terminal kinase/stress activated protein kinase (JNK/SAPK) (Weinstein et al, 1992). It was shown that a plant flavonoids, quercetin, inhibited inducible nitric oxide synthetase (iNOS) expression by inhibiting p38 MAPK (Wadsworth and Koop, 2001) and inhibited TNF-α -induction from LPS-induced RAW cells by inhibiting JNK/SAPK, leading to the inhibition of AP-1-DNA binding (Wadsworth et al, 2001). In a separate pathway, quercetin inhibited ERK 1/2 and p38 MAPK to regulate the post-transcriptional level of TNF-α. It has been shown that quercetin inhibited NF-B activation by ERK and p38 kinase inhibition (Cho et al, 2003). Another plant flavonoid, wogonin, inhibited monocyte chemotactic protein-1 gene expression of 12-O-tetradecanoylphorbol 13-acetate (TPA)-induced human endothelial cells by AP-1 repression through ERK 1/2 and JNK inhibition (Chang et al, 2001).

Studies have shown clearly that anti-inflammatory medicinal plants inhibited the expression of various inflammation-related proteins/enzymes, at least partly, by suppressing the activation of transcription factors such as NF-B and AP-1 (Kim et al, 2004). These suppressions might be mediated via inhibition of several protein kinases involved in the signal transduction pathway.

7.0   Some Nigerian Anti-inflammatory Herbs

The use of anti-inflammatory herbs for health improvement has a long and successful history in traditional medicine in Nigeria. Many herbal preparations are used to treat fever and inflammation in the traditional folklore medicine. The hope of discovering novel therapeutic agents capable of suppressing, reducing, or relieving pain as well as inflammation is high.

Many human and animal diseases, such as arthritic disorders, lupus erythematosus, asthma, bronchitis, inflammatory bowel disease, ulcerative colitis, pancreatitis, ascities, hepatitis, cancer and infections are associated with different degrees of inflammation. Even malaria and malaria fever have some inflammatory components (Perlmann and Troye-Blomberg, 2000 and the evidence in the body of the book). The infection of the liver and the red blood cells by the hepatic and erythrocytic plasmodia schizonts leads to severe inflammation of hepatocytes. The clinical manifestations of malaria, fever and chills, are associated with the synchronous rupture of the infected erythrocytes and the release of metabolites with potent proinflammtory activities (Perlmann and Troye-Blomberg, 2000). For this reason, antipyretic and anti-inflammatory therapies are often essential in the treatment of malaria. This could explain the benefits and instant relief experienced by malaria patients when they use anti-inflammatory medications, including some herbal medications with known antiphlogistic properties.

The treatment of rheumatic disorders (inflammation) is one area in which Nigerian traditional medical practitioners enjoy patronage and success. A good number of plant species are available for this purpose, and the method of usage differs from one area to another. Scientific evaluation of some of these plants, for instance, Mitracarpus scaber (Ekpendu, et al, 1994), Pavetta cressipes (Amos et al, 1998), Culcasia scadens (Okoli and Akah 2000, Akah and Okoli 2004), Asytasia gangetica (Akah et al 2003a), Aframomum melegueta (Okoli et al 2007), Afzelia Africana (Akah et al 2007), Spondias mombin (Nworu et al 2011) and Lupinus arboreus (Ohadoma et al 2011) among others have been reported. The most common practice involves taking the extracts orally as decoctions or infusions; washing the inflamed part (e.g. swollen knee) with the extracts; applying squeezed herb as poultice on inflamed part (Akah and Nwambie, 1994, Akah et al 2003b). Some other local medicinal plants which have been used in folklore medicine to treat inflammation, fever, and rheumatic ailments are shown in table 3.

Table 3. Some local medicinal plants used in folklore medicine to treat inflammation, rheumatism, and fever

Plant	Family	Parts of plant and reparation

Gymnema sylvestre	Asclepiadaceae	leaf
Acanthus montanus (Nees)	Acanthaceae	Infusion of leaves taken 3 times daily
Schwenka Americana Linn	Solanaceae	Whole plant; Crushed and used as poultice
Zanha golungensis Hiern	Sapindaceae	Leaves; Chopped fresh leaves applied on inflamed sores
Cardiospermum grandio Florum Swart	Sapindaceae	Whole plant; leaves mixed with castor oil and used orally to treat rheumatism and lumbago
Paullinia pinnata Linn	Sapindaceae	Boil leaves and drink as desired
Allophylus Africana P. Beauv	Sapindaceae	Bark, root, and leaves; boiled in water and used as tea
Achyranthes aspera Linn	Amaranthaceae	Whole plant; Boiled in water and used as tea
Cythula prostrate (L.) Blume	Amaranthaceae	Leaves; Crushed with alcohol and used as poultice
Alternanthera repens (L.) Kuntze	Amaranthaceae	Leaves; Decoction used as tea
Monodara myristica (Gaertn) Dumal	Annonaceae	Leaves and bark; Chopped fresh leaves applied on fresh sores
Ocimum basilicum Linn	Labiatae	Whole plant; Infusion drunk once daily
Entadrophragma cylindricum Sprague	Meliaceae	Bark; macerated in alcohol and used as a drink
Ekebergia senegalensis A. Juss	Meliaceae	Leaves; Infusion drunk as tea
Lecaniodiscus cupaniodes (Planch)	Sapindaceae	Roots and leaves; Extracts are taken orally for a long time for rheumatism and arthritis
Chassalia kolly (Schumach.) Heppner	Rubiaceae	Leaves; Extract of bark taken as tea
Securidaca longipedunculata Fres	Polygalaceae	Leaves and roots; Paste of root bark and leaves is applied externally on sores and to cure rheumatism

Strophanthus hispidus Oliv	Apocynaceae	Leaves; Decoction taken as tea
Astonia boonei De Wild	Apocynaceae	Leaves, sap, and stem bark; Topical application of the latex on the swollen part and leaf infusion drunk as desired
Funtumia Africana (Benth) Stapf.	Apocynaceae	Leaves; Decoction taken as tea
Abrus precatorius L.	Fabaceae	Leaves and stem; decoction and infusion are drunk
Ageratum conyzoides Linn	Asteraceae	Leaves and flowers; fresh leaves applied on fresh sores and infusion drunk
Tetrapleura tetraptera (taub)	Fabaceae	Fruits; decoction and infusion drunk
Alchornea cordifolia	Euphorbiaceae	Leaves; Ground leaves applied to wounds and aches
Aspillia Africana C.D. Adams	Compositae	Chopped leaves applied on inflamed sores
Combretum racemosum P. Beauv	Combretaceae	Leaves; Leaf infusion administered orally
Salacia pallescens Oliv	Celastraceae	Leaves; Crushed with alcohol and used as poultice
Desmodium triflorum DC	Papilionaceae	Whole plant; a powder is made and taken with pap
Plumbago zeylanica Linn	Plumbaginaceae	Roots and leaves; Decoction is drunk
Pepperomia pellucida L. HBK	Piperaceae	Aerial part; Squeezed juice used for eye inflammation and headaches
Anchomanes difformis Engl	Araceae	Aqueous decoction of the Rhizome taken orally
Anthocleista d'jalonensis A. Chev	Loganiaceae	Ethanol decoction of stem bark taken orally
Diodiu sarmentosa Swartz	Rubiaceae	Aqueous leaf extract taken orally and applied locally
Hexalobus monopetalous Engl	Anonaceae	Aqueous infusion of root bark extract taken orally

Mitracarpus scarber Zucc	Rubiaceae	Aqueous decoction of leaf extract taken orally
Morinda lucida Benth	Rubiaceae	Alcoholic infusion of leaf taken orally and applied externally
Palisota hirsuta K. Schum	Commelineceae	Aqueous infusion of leaf taken orally
Pentaclethra macrophylla Benth	Mimosaceae	Aqueous decoction of seed taken orally
Securidaca longipedunculata Fresen	Polygalaceae	Aqueous infusion of leaf taken orally and applied externally
Strophamus hispidus Oliv	Apocynaceae	Aqueous decoction of leaf extract taken orally

8.0   Conclusion

Inflammation acts as a central executor in the pathogenesis of many diseases such as rheumatoid arthritis, arteriosclerosis, myocarditis, infections, cancer, metabolic disorders, and many more. Monocytes and macrophages are the key players in inflammatory responses and are also the major sources of pro-inflammatory mediators and enzymes including tumour necrosis factor—a (TNF-α), interleukins (ILs), cyclooxygenase (COX), and nitric oxide synthase (NOS). These genes of pro-inflammatory mediators are strongly induced during inflammation and are responsible for its initiation and persistence. TNF- α and IL-1β are the cytokines that act as signalling molecules for immune cells and coordinate the inflammatory responses. Cyclooxygenase-2 (COX-2) is an enzyme which is necessary for the production of pro-inflammatory prostaglandins and thus has been a target for many present anti-inflammatory medicinal plants. Nitric oxide (NO) is a free radical that mediates many physiological and pathophysiological processes, including neurotransmission and inflammation. Expression of the inducible isoform of NOS (iNOS) in activated macrophages is mainly responsible for production of pathological concentration of NO during inflammation. Therefore suppression of iNO synthetase expression is an important target through which many anti-inflammatory medicinal plants mediate their activities. It is established that nuclear factor-κB (NF-κB) and AP-1 play the most important roles in the immune system. NF-κB is reported to regulate the expression of nearly all inflammatory mediators involved in inflammation. Nuclear translocation of NF- κB and AP-1 in response to various pro-inflammatory stimuli is associated with the activation of inflammatory cascade and therefore, these transcriptional factors are a primary target of many anti-inflammatory medicinal plants and their compounds.

Since anti-inflammatory medicinal plant extracts are usually multi-component, it is likely that they act on multiple targets to impact the complex equilibrium of whole cellular networks of immune cells. This could be more favourable than agents that act on a single target since complementary actions on many genes might be needed to modify inflammatory disease processes. In other words, the efficacy of herbal therapy and herb-based anti-inflammatory compounds might depend on the perturbation of more than one target.

References

Akah PA, Nwambie AI (1994). Evaluation of Nigerian traditional medicines: 1. Plants used for rheumatic (inflammatory) disorders, J. Ethnopharmacol. 42: 179-182.

Akah PA, Ezike AC, Nwafor SV, Okoli CO, Enwerem (2003a) Evaluation of the anti-asthmatic property of Asytasia gangetica leaf extracts. J.Ethnopharmacol. 89: 25-36.

Akah PA, Okoli CO, Nwafor SV (2003b). Anti-inflammatory plants J. Natr. Remed. 3: 1-30.

Akah PA, Okoli CO (2004). Mechanism of the anti-inflammatory activity of the leaf extract of Culcasia scandens.P. Baeuv (Araceae). Pharm. Biochem. Bev. 79: 473-481.

Akah PA, Okpi O, Okoli CO (2007). Evaluation of the anti-inflammatory, analgesic and antimicrobial activities of the bark of Afzelia Africana. Nig. J. Nat. Prod. Med. 11: 48-52.

Ammon HPT, Anazodo MI, Safayhi H, Dhawan BN, Srimal RC (1992). Curcumin: a potent inhibitor of leukotriene B4 formation in rat peritoneal polymorphonuclear neutrophils (PMNL). Planta Med 58: 226.

Amos S, Okwuasaba FK, Gamaniel K, Akah PA, Nwambebe C. Anti-inflammatory and muscle relaxant effects of aqueous extract of Pavetta cressipes leaves. Fitoterapia 69: 425-428.

Barbosa NR, Fischmann L, Talib LL, Gattaz WF (2004). Inhibition of platelet phospholipase A2 activity by catuaba extract suggests anti-inflammatory properties, Phytother Res. 18(11):942-944.

Barnes PJ (1998). Anti-inflammatory actions of glucocorticoids: molecular mechanisms. Clinical Science 94: 557-572.

Bauman J, Bruchhausen FV, Wurm G (1980). Flavonoids and related compounds as inhibitors of arachidonic acid peroxidation. Prostaglandins. 20:627-639.

Benrezzouk R, Terencio MC, Ferrandiz ML, Hernandez-Perez M, Rabanal R, Alcaraz MJ (2001). Inhibition of 5-lipoxygenase activity by the natural anti-inflammatory compound aethiopinone. Inflamm Res 50: 96-101.

Braga FC, Wagner H, Lombardi JA, Braga de Oliveira A (2000). Screening Brazilian plant species for in vitro inhibition of 5-lipoxygenase. Phytomedicine 6: 447-452.

Chan MM (1995). Inhibition of tumor necrosis factor by curcumin, a phytochemical. Biochem Pharmacol 49:1551-1556.

Chang CJ, Geahlen RL (1992). Protein-tyrosine kinase inhibition: mechanism-based discovery of antitumor agents. J Nat Prod. 55:1529-1590.

Chang YL, Shen JJ, Wung BS, Chen JJ, Wang DL (2001). Chinese herbal remedy wogonin inhibits monocyte chemotactic protein-1 gene expression in human endothelial cells. Mol Pharmacol. 60: 507-513.

Chen S (2011). Natural products triggering biological targets--a review of the anti-inflammatory phytochemicals targeting the arachidonic acid pathway in allergy asthma and rheumatoid arthritis. Curr Drug Target 12(3):288-301.

Cho KJ, Yun CH, Packer L, Chung AS (2001). Inhibition mechanisms of bioflavonoids extracted from the bark of Pinus maritima on the expression of pro-inflammatory cytokines. Ann N Y Acad Sci 928:141-156.

Cho SY, Park SJ, Kwon MJ, Jeong TS, Bok SH, Choi WY, Jeong WI, Ryu SY, Do SH, Lee CS, Song JC, Jeong KS (2003). Quercetin suppresses pro inflammatory cytokines production through MAP kinases and NF-?B pathway in lipopolysaccharide- stimulated macrophage. Mol Cell Biochem.243:153-160.

Cotrim CA, de Oliveira SC, Diz Filho EB, Fonseca FV, Baldissera L Jr, Antunes E, Ximenes RM, Monteiro HS, Rabello MM, Hernandes MZ, de Oliveira Toyama D, Toyama MH (2011). Quercetin as an inhibitor of snake venom secretory phospholipase A2. Chem Biol Interact. 89(1-2):9-16.

Coy-Barrera ED, Cuca-Suarez LE (2011). In vitro anti-inflammatory effects of naturally-occurring compounds from two Lauraceae plants. An Acad Bras Cienc. Oct 21. pii: S0001-37652011005000044.

Crofford LJ, Oates JC, McCune WJ, Gupta S, Kaplan MJ, Catella-Lawson F, Morrow JD, McDonagh KT, Schmaier AH (2000). Thrombosis in patients with connective tissue diseases treated with specific cyclooxygenase 2 inhibitors. A report of four cases. Arthritis Rheum. 43:1891-1896.

Davis L, Kuttan G (1999). Effect of Withania somnifera on cytokine production in normal and cyclophosphamide treated mice. Immunopharmacol Immunotoxicol 1999;21:695-703.

Dhuley JN (1997). Effect of some Indian herbs on macrophage functions in ochratoxin -A treated mice. J Ethnopharmacol 58:15-20.

Ekpendu TO, Akah PA, Adesomuju AA, Okogun JI (1994). Anti-inflammatory and anti-microbial activities of Mtracarpus scaber Int. J. Pharmacog.. 32: 191-196.

El Sohly H, Little T, El Sohly JR, El Sohly M. (1990). Canniprene: a prototype anti-inflammatory natural product. Planta Med 56: 662-663.

Ferrandiz ML, Ramachandran Nair AG, Alcaraz MJ (1990). Inhibition of sheep platelet arachidonate metabolism by flavonoids from Spanish and Indian medicinal herbs. Pharmazie. 45:206-208.

Ferriola PC, Cody V, Middleton E (1989). Protein kinase C inhibition by plant flavonoids. Kinetic mechanisms and structural-activity relationships. Biochem Pharmacol. 38:1617-1624.

Fiebich BL, Heinrich M, Hiller KO, Kammerer N (2001). Inhibition of TNF-alpha synthesis in LPS-stimulated primary human monocytes by Harpagophytum extract SteiHap 69. Phytomedicine 8:28-30.

Fujiki H, Suganuma M, Kurusu M, Okabe S, Imayoshi Y, Taniguchi S, Yoshida T (2003). New TNF-alpha releasing inhibitors as cancer preventive agents from traditional herbal medicine and combination cancer prevention study with EGCG and sulindac or tamoxifen. Mutat Res 523-524:119-125.

Fukuishi N, Takada T, Fukuyama Y, Akagi M (2001). Antiallergic effect of ardisiaquinone A: a potent 5-lipoxygenase inhibitor. Phytomedicine 8: 460-464.

Fukuyama Y, Kiriyama Y, Okino J, Kodama M, Iwaki H, Hosozawa S, Matsui K (1993). Naturally occuring 5-lipoxygenase inhibitor. II. Structures and syntheses of ardisianones A and B, and maesanin, alkenyl-1,4 benzoquinones from the rhizome of Ardisia japonica. Chem Pharm Bull 41: 561–565.

Giner-Larza EM, Máñez S, Recio MC, Giner RM, Prieto JM, Cerdá-Nicolás M, Ríos JL (2001). Oleanonic acid, a 3-oxotriterpene from Pistacia, inhibits leukotriene synthesis and has anti-inflammatory activity. Eur J Pharmacol 428: 137–143.

Giner-Larza EM, Máñez S, Giner RM, Recio MC, Prieto JM, Cerdá-Nicolás M, Ríos JL (2002). Anti-inflammatory triterpenes from Pistacia terebinthus Galls. Planta Med 68: 311–315.

Hidaka H, Ishiko T, Furuhashi T, Kamohara H, Suzuki S, Miyazaki M, Ikeda O, Mita S, Setoguchi T, Ogawa M (2002). Curcumin inhibits interleukin 8 production and enhances interleukin 8 receptor expression on the cell surface: impact on human pancreatic carcinoma cell growth by autocrine regulation. Cancer 95:1206-1214.

Hodge G, Hodge S, Han P (2002). Allium sativum (garlic) suppresses leukocyte inflammatory cytokine production in vitro: potential therapeutic use in the treatment of inflammatory bowel disease. Cytometry 48:209-215.

Hong T, Jin GB, Yoshino G, Miura M, Maeda Y, Cho S, Cyong JC (2002). Protective effects of Polygalae root in experimental TNBS-induced colitis in mice. J. Ethnopharmacol 79:341- 346.

Hsieh TC, Kunicki J, Darzynkiewicz Z, Wu JM (2002). Effects of extracts of Coriolus versicolor (I'm-Yunity) on cell-cycle progression and expression of interleukins-1 beta, -6, and -8 in promyelocytic HL-60 leukemic cells and mitogenically stimulated and nonstimulated human lymphocytes. J Alter Compl. Med 8: 591-602.

Huang KS, Lin M, Yu LN, Kong M (2000). Four novel oligostilbenes from the roots of Vitis amurensis. Tetrahedron 56: 1321–1329. Ihantola-Vormisto A, Summanen J, Kankaanranta H, Vuorela H, Asmawi ZM, Moilanen E. (1997). Anti-inflammatory activity of extracts from leaves of Phyllanthus emblica. Planta Med 63: 518-524.

Iizuka N, Miyamoto K, Hazama S, et al. (2000). Anticachectic effects of Coptidis rhizoma, an anti-inflammatory herb, on esophageal cancer cells that produce interleukin 6. Cancer Lett 158:35-41.

Ito M, Tchoua U, Okamoto M, Tojo H (2002). Purification and Properties of a Phospholipase A2/Lipase Preferring Phosphatidic Acid, Bis(monoacylglycerol) Phosphate, and Monoacylglycerol from Rat Testis J. Biol. Chem. 277(10): 43674-43681.

Jang DS, Cuendet M, Su BN, Totura S, Riswan S, Fong HH, Pezzuto JM, Kinghorn AD (2004). Constituents of the seeds of Hernandia ovigera with inhibitory activity against cyclooxygenase-2. Planta Med. 70(10):893-896.

Jiang J, Xu Q (2003). Immunomodulatory activity of the aqueous extract from rhizome of Smilax glabra in the later phase of adjuvant-induced arthritis in rats. J. Ethnopharmacol 85:53-59.

Kammoun M, Miladi S, Ben Ali Y, Damak M, Gargouri Y, Bezzine S (2011). In vitro study of the PLA2 inhibition and antioxidant activities of Aloe vera leaf skin extracts. Lipids Health Dis. 11:10:30.

Kang JM, Kim N, Kim B, Kim JH, Lee BY, Park JH, Lee MK, Lee HS, Jang IJ, Kim JS, Jung HC, Song IS (2009). Gastroprotective action of Cochinchina momordica seed extract is mediated by activation of CGRP and inhibition of cPLA(2)/5-LOX pathway. Dig Dis Sci. 54(12):2549-2560.

Khanapure SP, Garvey DS, Janero DR, Letts LG (2007). Eicosanoids in inflammation: biosynthesis, pharmacology, and therapeutic frontiers. Curr Top Med Chem. 7(3): 311-340.

Kim HM, Lee EH, Na HJ, Lee SB, Shin TY, Lyu YS, Kim NS, Nomura S (1998). Effect of Polygala tenuifolia root extract on the tumor necrosis factor-alpha secretion from mouse astrocytes. J Ethnopharmacol 61:201-208.

Kim HM, Park YA, Lee EJ, Shin TY (1999). Inhibition of immediate-type allergic reaction by Rosa davurica Pall. in a murine model. J Ethnopharmacol 67:53-60.

Kim HP, Son KH, Chang HW, Kang SS (2004). Anti-inflammatory Plant Flavonoids and Cellular Action Mechanisms. J Pharmacol Sci 96: 229-245.

Kim YH, Ko WS, Ha MS, Lee CH, Choi BT, Kang HS, Kim HD (2000). The production of nitric oxide and TNF-alpha in peritoneal macrophages is inhibited by Dichroa febrifuga Lour. J Ethnopharmacol 69:35-43.

Kim YH, Ko WS, Ha MS, Lee CH, Choi BT, Kang HS, Kim HD (2000). The production of nitric oxide and TNF-alpha in peritoneal macrophages is inhibited by Dichroa febrifuga Lour. J Ethnopharmacol 69:35-43.

Krol W, Czuba ZP, Threadgill MD, Cunningham BD, Pietse G (1995). Inhibition of nitric oxide (NO) production in murine macrophages by flavones. Biochem Pharmacol. 50:1031-1035.

Kumar S, Ziereis K, Wiegrebe W, Müller K (2000). Medicinal plants from Nepal: evaluation as inhibitors of leukotriene biosynthesis. J Ethnopharmacol 70: 191-195.

Kumari R, Meyyappan A, Selvamani P, Mukherjee J, Jaisankar P (2011). Lipoxygenase inhibitory activity of crude bark extracts and isolated compounds from Commiphora berryi. J Ethnopharmacol. 31:138(1):256-259.

Kundu JK, Mossanda KS, Na HK, Surh YJ (2005). Inhibitory effects of the extracts of Sutherlandia frutescens (L.) R. Br. and Harpagophytum procumbens (Devil's Claw) on phorbol ester-induced COX-2 expression in mouse skin: AP-1 and CREB as potential upstream targets. Cancer Lett. 218(1):21-31.

Duo YC, Sun CM, Tsai WJ, Ou JC, Chen WP, Lin CY (1999). Blocking of cellproliferation, cytokines production and genes expression following administration of Chinese herbs in the human mesangial cells. Life Sci 64:2089-2099.

Lanni C, Becker EL (1985). Inhibition of neutrophil phospholipase A2 by p-bromophenylacyl bromide, nordihydroguaiaretic acid, 5,8,11,14-eicosatetrayenoic acid and quercetin. Int Archs Allergy Appl Immun. 76:214-217.

Laughton MJ, Evans PJ, Moroney MA, Hoult JRS, Halliwell B (1991). Inhibition of mammalian 5-lipoxygenase and cyclooxygenase by flavonoids and phenolic dietary additives. Biochem Pharmacol. 42:1673-1681.

Lee HT, Yang SW, Kim KH, Seo EK, Mar W (2002). Pseudoguaianolides isolated from Inula britannica var. chinenis as inhibitory constituents against inducible nitric oxide synthase. Arch. Pharmacol Res 25: 151-153.

Lee T-P, Matteliano ML, Middletone E (1982). Effect of quercetin on human polymorphonuclear leukocyte lysosomal enzyme release and phospholipid metabolism. Life Sci. 31:2765-2774.

Lemaire I, Assinewe V, Cano P, Awang DV, Arnason JT (1999). Stimulation of interleukin-1 and -6 production in alveolar macrophages by the neotropical liana, Uncaria tomentosa (una de gato). J Ethnopharmacol 64:109-115.

Lindahl M, Tagesson C (1993). Selective inhibition of group II phospholipase-A2 by quercetin. Inflammation. 17:573-582.

Matsunaga K, Takahashi A, Ohizumi Y (2000). Inhibitory action of Paraguayan medicinal plants on 5-lipoxygenase. Nat Med 54: 151-154.

McMurray RW, Hardy KJ (2002). COX-2 inhibitors: today and tomorrow. Am J Med Sci. 323:181-189.

Momin RA, De Witt DL, Nair MG (2003). Inhibition of cyclooxygenase (COX) enzymes by compounds from Daucus carota L. Seeds. Phytother Res.17(8):976-979.

Moncada S, Palmer RMJ, Higgs EA (1991). Nitric oxide: physiology, pathophysiology, and pharmacology. Pharmacol Rev. 43:109-142.

Mollace V, Muscoli C, Masini E, Cuzzocrea S, Salvemini D (2005). Modulation of prostaglandin biosynthesis by nitric oxide and nitric oxide donors. Pharmacol Rev. 57(2):217-252.

Müller K, Ziereis K, Paper DH. 1998. Ilex aquifolium: Protection against enzymatic and non-enzymatic lipid peroxidation. Planta Med 64: 536-540.

Müller-Jakic B, Breu W, Pröbstle A, Redl K, Greger H, Bauer R (1994). In vitro inhibition of cyclooxygenase and 5-lipoxygenase by alkamides from Echinacea and Achillea species. Planta Med 60: 37-40.

Murakami M, Kudo I (2004). Recent advances in molecular biology and physiology of the prostaglandin E2-biosynthetic pathway. Prog Lipid Res. 43:30-35.

Nathan C (1992). Nitric oxide as a secretory product of mammalian cells. FASEB J. 6:3051-3064.

Needleman P, Isakson P (1997). The discovery and function of COX-2. J Rheumatol. 24 Suppl 49:6-8.

Newton R (2000). Molecular mechanisms of glucocorticoid action: what is important?" Thorax 55 (7): 603-613.

Nworu CS, Akah PA, Okoye FBC, Kamdem Toukam D, Udeh J, Esimone CO (2011). The leaf extract of Spondias mombin L. displays an anti-inflammatory effect and suppresses inducible formation of tumor necrosis factor-α and nitric oxide (NO). J. Immunotoxicol 8(01): 10-16.

Oh GS, Pae HO, Choi BM, Jeong S, Oh H, Oh CS, Rho YD, Kim DH, Shin MK, Chung HT (2003). Inhibitory effects of the root cortex of Paeonia suffruticosa on interleukin-8 and macrophage chemoattractant protein-1 secretions in U937 cells. J Ethnopharmacol 84:85-89.

Ohadoma SC, Akah PA, Nkemmele CA, Nnatuanya I, Nwosu PJC (2011). Investigation of the analgesic and anti-inflammatory activities of methanol leaf extract of Lupinus arboreus. J. Appl. Scs.14 : 10158-10169.

Okoli CO, Akah PA (2000). A pilot evaluation of the anti-inflammatory activity of Culcasia scandens, a traditional anti-rheumatic agent. J. Altern. Compl. Med. 6: 632-637.

Okoli CO, Akah PA, Nwafor SV, Ihemelandu UU, Amadife C (2007). Anti-inflammatory activity of seed extracts of Aframomum melegueta. J. Herbs Spices Med. Plants 13: 11-21.

Perlmann P, Troye-Blomberg M (2000). Malaria blood-stage infection and its control by the immune system. Folia biologica 46 (6): 210–218.

Ryu SY, Oak MH, Yoon SK, Cho DI, Yoo GS, Kim TS, Kim KM (2000). Anti allergic and anti-inflammatory triterpenes from the herb of Prunella vulgaris. Planta Med. 66: 358-360.

Sandoval M, Okuhama NN, Zhang XJ, Condezo LA, Lao J, Angeles' FM, Musah RA, Bobrowski P, Miller MJ (2002) Anti-inflammatory and antioxidant activities of cat's claw (Uncaria tomentosa and Uncaria guianensis) are independent of their alkaloid content. Phytomedicine 9: 325-337.

Schubert SY, Lansky EP, Neeman I (1999). Antioxidant and eicosanoid enzyme inhibition properties of pomegranate seed oil and fermented juice flavonoids. J Ethnopharmacol 66: 11–17.

Sendl A, Elbl G, Steinke B, Redl K, Breu W, Wagner H (1992). Comparative pharmacological investigations of Allium ursinum and Allium sativum. Planta Med 58: 1–6.

Shah BN, Seth AK, Maheshwari KM (2011). A Review on Medicinal Plants as a Source of Anti-inflammatory Agents. Res. J. Med. Plant, 5: 101-115.

Shon YH, Kim JH, Nam KS (2002). Effect of Astragali radix extract on lipopolysaccharide-induced inflammation in human amnion. Biol Pharm Bull 25:77-80.

Spellman K (2006). Modulation of cytokine expression by traditional medicines: a review of herbal immunomodulators. Altern. Med. Rev. 11(12): 128-150.

Stavri M, Ford CH, Bucar F, Streit B, Hall ML (2005). Bioactive constituents of Artemisia monosperma. Phytochemistry 66: 233-239.

Stuehr DJ (1999). Mammalian nitric oxide synthases. Biochim. Biophys. Acta 1411 (2-3): 217-230.

Su BN, Jones WP, Cuendet M, Kardono LB, Ismail R, Riswan S, Fong HH, Farnsworth NR, Pezzuto JM, Kinghorn AD (2004). Constituents of the stems of Macrococculus pomiferus and their inhibitory activities against cyclooxygenases-1 and -2. Phytochemistry. Nov;65(21):2861-2866.

Sunil Kumar KC, Müller K. (1998). Inhibition of leukotriene biosynthesis and lipid peroxidation in biological models by the extract of Cassia fistula. Phytother Res 12: 526-528.

Tornhamre S, Schmidt TJ, Näsman-Glaser B, Ericsson I, and Lindgreen JA (2001). Inhibitory effects of helenalin and related compounds on 5-Lipoxygenase and leukotriene C4 synthase in human blood cells. Biochem Pharmacol 62: 903-911.

Venema RC , Ju H, Zou R, Ryan JW, Venema VJ (1997). Subunit Interactions of Endothelial Nitric-oxide Synthase. J Biol Chem 272(2): 1276-1282.

Vane J, Botting (1987). Inflammation and the mechanism of action of anti-inflammatory drugs, The FASEB J. 1:89-96.

Wadsworth TL, Koop DR (2001). Effects of Ginkgo biloba extract (EGb 761) and quercetin on lipopolysaccharide-induced release of nitric oxide. Chem Biol Interact. 137:43-58.

Wadsworth TL, McDonald TL, Koop DR (2001). Effects of Ginkgo biloba extract (EGb 761) and quercetin on lipopolysaccharideinduced signaling pathways involved in the release of tumor necrosis factor-α. Biochem. Pharmacol. 62:963-974.

Wagner H (1989). Search for new plant constituents with potential antiphlogistic and anti-allergic activity. Planta Med 55: 235-241.

Wagner H, Dorsch W, Bayer Th, Breu W, Willer F (1990). Antiasthmatic effects of onions: inhibition of 5-lipoxygenase and cyclooxygenase in vitro by thiosulfinates and 'cepaenes'. Prostaglandins Leukot Essent Fatty Acids 39: 59-62.

Weinstein SL, Sanghera JS, Lemke K, DeFranco AL, Pelech SL (1992). Bacterial lipopolysaccharide induces tyrosine phosphorylation and activation of mitogen-activated protein kinases in macrophages. J Biol Chem. 267:14955-14962.

Welton AF, Tobias LD, Fiedler-Nagy C, Anderson W, Hope W, Meyers K, Coffey JW (1986). Effect of flavonoids on arachidonic acid metabolism. In: Cody V, Middleton E, Harborne JB, editors. Plant flavonoids in biology and medicine. New York: Alan R. Liss; p. 231-242.

Werz O (2007). Inhibition of 5-Lipoxygenase Product Synthesis by Natural Compounds of Plant Origin. Planta Med 73(13): 1331-1357.

358 Appendix 2

Yang LK, Khoo-Beattie, Goh KL (2001). Ardisiaquinones from Ardisia teysmanniana. Phytochemistry 58: 1235-1238.

Zalewski CA, Passero LF, Melo AS, Corbett CE, Laurenti MD, Toyama MH, Toyama DO, Romoff P, Fávero OA, Lago JH (2011). Evaluation of anti-inflammatory activity of derivatives from aerial parts of Baccharis uncinella. Pharm Biol. 49(6):602-607.

Zhao Z, Liu N, Huang J, Lu PH, Xu XM (2011). Inhibition of cPLA2 activation by Ginkgo biloba extract protects spinal cord neurons from glutamate excitotoxicity and oxidative stress-induced cell death. J Neurochem. 116(6):1057-1065.doi: 10.1111/j.1471-4159.2010.07160.x.

Wiart C (2006). Anti-inflammatory plants In: Ethnopharmacology of Medicinal Plants: Asia and the Pacific; Christopher Wiart (Ed.); Humana Press Inc., Totowa, NJ.

BIBLIOGRAPHY

Adeloye, Adelola, African Pioneers of Modern Medicine. Nigerian doctors of the nineteenth century, Ibadan, University Press Ltd, 1985.

Ademuwagun, J., A. A. Ayoade, I. E. Harrison and D. M. Warren, editors, African Therapeutic Systems, Boston, Cross Roads Press, 1979.

Ajayi, O.O. & D.T. Okpako, Prostaglandin-like substances in Burkitt's lymphoma tissue. British Journal of Cancer 1977 (36).

Albert, Adrian. Selective Toxicity. The physico-chemical basis of therapy, London, Chapman and Hall, 1951.

Alder, H.M. and V.B.O. Hammett, The doctor-patient relationship revisited: an analysis of the placebo effect. Annals of Internal Medicine. 1973, (78).

Andah, B.W. The oral versus the written word in the cognitive revolution: languages, culture and literacy. West African Journal of Anthropo-logy (WAJA) Special Book Issue, 1990 (20).

Apata, L The practice of herbalism in Nigeria. in: African Medicinal Plants, A. Sofowora, editor, Ile-Ife: University of Ife Press, 1979.

Atta, Ed. B. The pathology of sickle cell disease, in: Sickle-Cell Disease, A handbook for the general clinician, A.F. Fleming, editor, Churchill Livingstone, Edinburgh, 1982.

Barnes, P.J. Pathophysiology of asthma. British Journal of Clinical Pharmacology 1996, 42 (1).

Beecher, H.K. Surgery as placebo: a quantitative study of bias, Journal of the American Medical Association 1961, (176).

Bell, A.S. and L.C. Ranford-Cartwright. A real-time PCR assay for quantifying Plasmodium falciparum infections in the mosquito vector. International Journal of Parasitology 2004 (34).

Benson, H. and M.D. Epstein, The placebo effect: A neglected asset in the care of patients. Journal of the American Medical Association 1975 (232).

359

Benson, H. and D.P. McCallie Jr. Angina pectoris and the placebo effect. New England Journal of Medicine 1979 (300).

Blalock, J.C. Shared ligands and receptors as a molecular mechanism of communication between the immune and neuro-endocrine systems, Annals of the New York Academy of Science 1994 (741).

Braithwaite, E.K. The African presence in Caribbean literature. Daedalus Journal of the American Academy of Arts and Science, Cambridge, Harvard University Press, 1974.

Briskman, L Doctors and witch doctors, which doctors are which? British Medical Journal 1987, (295).

Bynum, W.F. An Early History of the British Pharmacological Society. London, British Pharmacological Society, 1981.

Chan, K. Traditional Chinese Medicine, Trends in Pharmacological Sciences 1995, (16).

Charles, R. Mind, Body and Immunity, How to enhance your body's natural defences, London, Methuen, 1990.

Chow, E.P.Y. Traditional Chinese medicine: a holistic system. in: Alternative Medicines, Popular and Policy Perspectives, W. Salmon, editor, New York & London, Tavistock, 1984.

Cirino, G. , S. Fiorucci and W.C. Sessa, Endothelial nitric oxide synthase: the cinderella of inflammation? Trends in Pharmacological Sciences 2003 (24).

Clark, Ian, Alison C. Budd, Lisa M Allevaand William B. Cowden, Human malaria disease: a consequence of inflammatory cytokine release, Malaria Journal 2006 (5).

Clark, I. A. & K.A. Rockett. Nitric oxide and parasitic disease, Advances in Parasitology 1996 (37).

Clark, I.A., K.A. Rockett and W.B. Cowden Annals Tropical Medicine Parasitology 1996 (90).

Contri, B., I. Tabarean, C. Andrei and T. Bafai, Cytokines and fever, Frontiers in Bioscience 2004 (9).

Davidson, Basil The Black Man's Burden–Africa and the Curse of the Nation-State, New York, Times Books, 1992.

Edozien, J. C. The serum proteins of healthy adult Nigerians. Journal of Clinical Pathology 1957 (10).

Edozien, J. C., Boyo, A. E. & Morley, D. C. The relationship of serum gamma-globulin concentration to malaria and sickling. Journal of Clinical Pathology 1960, (13).

Erhueh A.O. Vatican II: Image of God in Man, Urbaniana University Press, Rome, 1987.

Ernst, E. Homeopathy, a "helpful placebo" or an unethical intervention? Trends in Pharmacological Sciences 2010 (31).

Ernst, E. No to placebo effect. The Guardian (London) 22 February 2010.

Evans-Pritchard, E. E. Witchcraft, Oracles and Magic among the Azande, London, Oxford University Press, 1937.

Eysenck, H. J. Crime and Personality, St Albans, Paladin Frogmore Press, 1970.

Fleming, A. F. Sickle-cell trait. genetic counseling, in: Sickle Cell Disease, A Handbook for the General Clinician, A.F. Fleming, editor, Churchill Livingstone, London, 1982.

Frankel, S. The Huli Response to Illness, Cambridge, Cambridge University Press, 1986.

Fraser, J.G. The Fear of the Dead in Primitive Religion, London, Mac-millan & Co. 1933.

Fraser, T.R. On the characters, actions and therapeutical uses of the bean of Calabar (Physostigma venenosum, Balfour). Edinburgh Medical Journal, 1863 (9).

Galdini, R.B. Influence, Harper, 2007.

Gilles, Eva, E. E. Evans-Pritchard. Witchcraft, Oracles, and Magic among the Azande, Oxford, Clarendon Press, 1976.

Holmstedt, B. and J.G. Bruhn, Is there a place for ethnopharmacology in our time? Trends in Pharmacological Sciences 1982, (3).

Horton, R. African traditional thought and Western science, in: Rationality, B. R. Wilson, editor, Blackwell, 1976.

Horton, Robin and Ruth Finnegan, editors, Horton, Levy-Bruhl, Durkheim and the scientific revolution, in: Modes of Thought—essays on thinking in western and non-western societies, London, Faber & Faber, 1973.

Horton, R. Patterns of Thought in Africa and the West, Cambridge, Cambridge University Press, 1993.

Illich, Ivan, Medical Nemesis: the expropriation of health, London, Calder and Boyers, 1975.

Imperatto, P..J. African Folklore Medicine Practices and Beliefs of the Bambara and other Peoples, Baltimore, New York Press, 1977.

Isawumi, M. Yoruba system of plant nomenclature and its implications in traditional medicine. Nigerian Field 1990 (55).

Isoun, T.T. Evolution of Science and Technology in Nigeria, The experience of the Rivers State University of Science and Technology, Riverside Communications, Port Harcourt, 1978.

Izzo, A. A. & F. Capasso, Herbal medicine, cancer prevention and cyclooxygenas-2 inhibition, Trends in Pharmacological Sciences, 2003 (24).

Janzen, J. M. The Quest for Therapy: medical pluralism in the Lower Zaire. Berkeley, University of California Press, 1978.

Kleinman, A. Concepts and a model for the comparison of medical systems as cultural systems, in: Concepts of Health, Illness and Disease, Caroline Currer and Margaret Stacey, editors, Oxford, Bergamon Press, 1993.

Kuhn, T. S. The Structure of Scientific Revolution, 3rd ed, Chicago, University of Chicago Press, 1996.

Lambo, J.O. The healing power of herbs, with special reference to obstetrics and gynaecology. in: Medicinal Plants and Traditional Medicine in Africa, A. Sofowora, editor, John Wiley and Sons Limited, Cichester, 1982.

Lambo, T. A. Traditional African cultures and western medicine, in: Medicine and Culture, F N Poynter, editor, London, Wellcome Institute of the History of Medicine, 1969.

Lancaster Jr, J. R. Sickle ell disease: loss of the blood's WD40? Trends in Pharmacological Sciences 2003 (24).

Last, M. The professionalization of African medicine: Ambiguities and definitions. in: The Professionalisation of African Medicine. M. Last and G. L. Chavunduka, editors, Manchester, Manchester University Press, 1986.

Lex, Barbara, Voodoo death: New thoughts on an old explanation. American Anthropologist 1974 (76).

Lyon, M. L. Order and healing: The concept of order and its importance in the conceptualisation of healing. Medical Anthropology 1990 (12).

Luzzatto, L. Genetics of red cells and susceptibility to malaria. Blood 1979 (54).

Luzzatto, L., O Sodeinde & G. Martini, Genetic variation in the host and adaptive phenomena in Plasmodium falciparum infection, p. 159-173. in: Malaria and the Red Cell, London, Pitman,1983.

Luzzatto, L. Glucose-6-phosphate-dehydrogenase and other genetic factors interacting with drugs. in: Ethnic Differences in

Reaction to Drugs and Xenobiotics, Werner Kalow, H. Werner Goedde, Dharam P. Agarwal, editors, New York, Alan R. Liss, 1986.

Maclean U. Choices of treatment among the Yoruba. in: Culture and Curing, Perspectives on traditional medical beliefs and practices, P. Morley and R. Willis, editors, London, Peter Owen Ltd, 1978.

Maegraith, B. G. Pathological Processes in Malaria and Blackwater Fever, Oxford, Scientific Publications, 1948.

Makinde, M.A. Awo. The Last Conversation, Ibadan, Evans Brothers, 2010.

Man, S., W.Gao, C. Wei, and C. Liu, Anticancer drugs from traditional toxic Chinese medicines, Phyotherapy Research 2012 (26).

Mead, Margaret. Growing Up in New Guinea, London, Penguin Books, 1942.

Meurs, H. Maarsingh & J. Zaagsma, Arginase and asthma: novel insights into nitric oxide homeostasis and airway hyper-responsiveness Trends in Pharmacological Sciences 2003 (24).

Moerman, D.E. Physiology and Symbols: the anthropological implications of the placebo effect, in: L. Romanucci-Ross, D.E. Moerman and L.R. Tancredi, editors, The Anthropology of Medicine, New York, Praeger, 1983.

Morris, B. Anthropological Studies of Religion: An introductory text, Cambridge, Cambridge University Press, 1995.

Nabofa, M.Y.and B.O. Elugbe, Epha: An Urhobo system of divination and its esoteric language. in: Studies in Urhobo Culture, P. Ekeh, editor, Urhobo Historical Society, Monograph No. 2, 2005.

Obeyesekere, G. The theory of psychological medicine in the Ayuverdic tradition, Culture, Medicine and Psychiatry 1977 (1).

Oduola, A., M.J., Sowunmi, A. Milhouse, W.R., Kyle, D.E. Martin, S. K. Walker and L.A. Salako, Innate resistance to new antimarial drugs in P. falciparum from Nigeria. Transactions Royal Society Tropical Medicine & Hygiene 1991 (84).

BIBLIOGRAPHY

Ogunniyi, M.B. Traditional African culture and modern science, in: Nigeria since Independence: the first 25 years, vol VII, Peter Ekeh and Garba Asiwaju, editors, Ibadan, Heineman Educational Books, 1989.

Okpako, D.T. Good Drugs Don't Grow on Trees or Do They? Ibadan, Ibadan University Press, 1988.

Okpako, D.T. Principles of Pharmacology - a tropical approach Cambridge, Cambridge University Press, 1991; second edition 2003.

Okpako, D.T. Traditional African medicine: Theory and pharmacology explored. Trends in Pharmacologica Sciences 1999 (20).

Okpako, D.T. Malaria and Indigenous Knowledge in Africa, Ibadan, Ibadan University Press, 2011.

Oliver-Bever, B. Medicinal Plants in Tropical West Africa, Cambridge, Cambridge University Press, 1986.

Osuntokun, B. O. The traditional basis of neuropsychiatric practice among the Yoruba of Nigeria. Tropical and Geographical Medicine 1975 (27).

Pearce, J.M.S. The placebo enigma, Quarterly Journal Medicine 1995, (88).

Popper, K. R. The Logic of Scientific Discovery, 8th impression, London, Hutchinson, 1975.

Price-Williams, D.R. A case study of ideas concerning disease among the Tiv. in: African Therapeutic Systems. Z.A. Ademuwagen, J.A. Ayoade, I.E. Harrison, and D.M. Warren, editors, Boston, Crossroads Press, 1979.

Rang, H.P., M.M. Dale & J.M. Ritter, Pharmacology 4th ed. Edinburgh, Churchill Livingstone,1999.

Rivers, W. H. R. Medicine, Magic and Religion, New York, Kegan Paul, Trench, Trubner and Company, 1924.

Ross, P. Homeopathy, a helpful placebo or an unethical intervention? Edzard Ernst Reply, Trends in Pharmacological Sciences 2010 (31).

Routledge, P. Murder, mystery, medicine and their practitioners, Pharmacology Matters /Newsletter (August 2011).

Sawyerr, H. An inquiry into some aspects of psychic influence in African understanding of life, in: Themes in African Social and Political Thought. O Otite, editor, Enugu, Fourth Dimension Publishers, 1978.

Sears, Cathy. The chimpanzee's medicine chest. New Scientist 4 August 1990 (127).

Selye, H. The Stress of Life, New York, McGraw-Hill Book Co, 1978.

Shellard, E.J. The significance of research into medicinal plants. in: A. Sofowora, editor, African Medicinal Plants. Proceedings, Pan African Conference on Research into Medicinal Plants, at the University of Ife, Ile-Ife in April 1974; University of Ife Press, Ile-Ife, Nigeria 1979.

Silverman, D.P. Divinity and deities in ancient Egypt, in: Religion in Ancient Egypt, B. E. Schafer, editor, London, Rutledge, 1991.

Sofowora, A. Medicinal Plants and Traditional Medicine in Africa John Wiley and Sons Limited, Cichester, 1982

Sogolo, G. Foundations of African Philosophy--A definitive analysis of conceptual issues in African thought. Ibadan, Ibadan University Press, 1993.

Stautgart, F. Traditional health care in Botswana. in: Professionalization of African Medicine. M. Last and G. L. Chavunduka, editors, Manchester, Manchester University Press, 1986.

Straub, H. R. Complexity of the bi-directional neuro-immune junction in the spleen, Trends in Pharmacological Sciences 2004 (25).

Subbaramaiah, K. & A.J. Dannenberg, Cyclooxygenase 2: a molecular target for cancer prevention and treatment Trends in Pharmacological Sciences 2003 (24).

Tavener, J. Primordial depth, in: BBC Belief, Jane Blakewell, editor, London, Duckworth Overlook, 2005.

Thomas, M. The Ayurvedic system of medicine, in: Principles of Pharmacology: tropical approach, second edition, DT Okpako, editor, Cambridge, Cambridge University Press, 2003.

Turner, V. Drums of Affliction - A study of religious processes among the Ndemu of Zambia. London, IAP Hutchinson University for Africa, 1981.

Twumasi, P.A. Medical systems in Ghana-A study in medical sociology Tema, Ghana Publishing Corporation, 1975.

Ukoli, F.M.A. Order among Parasites, Inaugural lecture, Ibadan University Press, University of Ibadan 1974.

Verger, Pierre Fatumbi, Ewe, the use of Plants in Yoruba Society, Sao Palo, Brazil, Odebrecht, 1995.

Vlachojannis, J. F. Magora, S. Chrubasik, Willow species and aspirin: different mechanisms of action, Phytotherapy and Research 2011 (25).

Weggen, S., M. Rogers & J. Erikson, NSAIDs: small molecules for the prevention of Alzheimer's disease or precursors for future drug development? Trends in Pharmacological Sciences 2007 (28).

Williamson, E.M., D.T. Okpako, Fred Evans, Pharmacological Methods in Phytotherapy Research, John Wiley & Sons, New York, 1996.

Wiredu, K. Philosophy and an African Culture, Cambridge, Cambridge University Press, 1980.

Work, T. S. & E. Work,The Basis of Chemotherapy, Oliver and Boyd, Edinburgh, 1948.

World Health Organization, African Traditional Medicine, Regional Office for Africa, Brazzaville, Afro Technical Report Series Number 1, 1976; also see www.WHO.int/medicines/areas /traditional/definitions/en (accessed 15 December 2014).

INDEX

Adeloye, Adelola
  attitudes of western-trained physicians to traditional African medicine, 33-34, 252
Ademuwagun, Zack
  on taboos and preventive medicine, 139
Akinkugbe, Professor O.O.
  on herbalists measuring hypertension, 271
akuobisi tree
  sacred among the Edo people, 201-202
ancestor spirit anger belief, 2, 4, 16, 17,47, 49, 50,53-54,58-59,61-65, 64-65, 70, 73, 81, 83, 85-90,92-94 320
  and the moral cohesion of the clan, 5-6, 17, 105, 107-108
  immorality and death, 107
  as a scientific theory, 61,63-65, 77
  as superstition, 65, 77
  as a metaphor, 72-74, 82
  steps in appeasing ancestor anger, 73
  divination and confession, 53, 73-74, 104-105
  an esoteric practice in TAM [153], 4, 7, 12
ancestor anger and illness
  moral issues, 7
  belief that ancestor anger can

cause illness, 2, 4, 6, 48, 71
  and the disruption of harmonious clan relations, 5-6, 17, 46, 71, 105, 107-108
  and psychoneuroimmuno-logy, 4, 73
  as a scientific theory, 63-64, 72-73, 79, 100-101
  holistic approach to disease, 77
anti-inflammatory plants, 121, 122, 271
  and the rat paw inflammation model experiment, 271
  common knowledge in most African households, 273
  see appendix 2, for a review of, 327
Apata, Chief Labulo
  traditional healer, 118
Awolowo, Chief Obafemi
  views on magun, 143-144
Ayurveda, (traditional Indian medicine)
  a long history of written documentation, 42-43
  and the harmony of the three doshas, 42-43
Azande (Sudanese) [also see Pritchard]
  witchcraft among, 65-67, 145
Calabar bean [also see etu esere]
  anti-cholinesterase properties of, 170, 171

---

[153]TAM= traditional African medicine

367

cancer
> inflammation and the cyclooxygenase-2 (COX-2), 287
> and Burkitt's lymphoma, 287-287-288

Chinese traditional medicine,
> and the restoration of harmony through ying and yang, 43

curse (the)
> the power and potency of,148-149

cytokine factor in inflammation/fever, 278-280, 304

Dale,Henry and Otto Loewi
> share Nobel prize on eserine,176, 178

disease and stress, 99-100

dosage in traditional African medicine, 129, 161, 166, 211, 213-214, 246

Durkheim, Emil
> non literate people and scientific thinking, 48-40

Elugbe, Ben
> and Urhobo divination, 130-131, 133

emuerinvwin (Urhobo)
> immoral or antisocial act and illness, 2, 102
> and ancestor anger, 1-2,
>> linked to chronic disease among individuals, 4, 72, 82, 87-88
>> and confession of immoral behaviour, 88, 89, 92
> literal meaning of, 83
> case histories of, 89-95
> incest, 3-4, 58, 88
> importance of mental harm-ony and good health, 45

relevance to universal health, 98

Erinvwin
> spiritual location of dead ancestors, 54
> categories of dead ancestors, 56-57
> moral force in the society, 58-59
> high ranking ancestors, 57, 59 70
> relationship to serious illness and death, 88, 96, 97, 98
> and troubled conscience, 99

Ernst, Edzard
> on homeopathy, 235-236

eserine
> from Physostigma veneno-sum, 168
> and structural elucidation, 171
> molecular structure, 171-172
> and Dale and Loewi shared Nobel prize, 176, 178
> research by Dale, 176-178
> and research by Otto Loewi
>> on vagus nerve stimula-tion, 176-178
> and theory of neurohumoral transmission, 178

etu esere bean of Calabar, 167-181
> used to identify witches, 167, 168, 172-174
> how the drug works, 173-175
> and Efik/Ibibio people, 167, 179
>> Akwa Ibom, 168
>> Cross River, 168
> physostigmine, properties of, 168
> T.R. Fraser and medical potential of, 167, 169-171

European traditional medicine
Hippocrates, 44
Galen, 44
Paraclesus, 44
Evans-Pritchard, Edward
on traditional African medicine, 18
on witchcraft among the Azande, 65-66, 145, 174-175
dosage
traditional plant remedies, 161
and poisonous plants, 160-161, 163, 164
no specific measurement in TAM, 161, 248
modern medicine targets the specific disease, 220, 281, 293
divination
role of traditional healing practices, 192, 213, 220, 228-229, 231, 247, 269
fever
and traditional healing systems, 8, 9, 19, 68, 267-273
a pharmacopoeia of anti-inflammatory plants in TAM, 20, 271
and TAM treatment of malaria, 247- 265
a key indicator of illness, 280,
Fleming, A.F.
president, Nigerian Sickle Cell Society, 263
and children with Hb-AS, 262, 263, 291, 303-304
Fraser, T.R.
and Calabar ordeal by poison, 168- 170
and anti-cholinesterase properties of the Calabar bean, 170-171
germ theory of disease, 121, 166, 220
established in late 19th century, 44
exponents of: Pasteur, Lister, Koch, and Erlich, 44
and harmony with humours, 44
glaucoma medicine
from the Calabar esere bean, 167-181
Glucose-6-phosphate dehydrogenase (G6PD), 256, 258
deficiency in Nigerians from birth, 256, 258, 303
and Plasmodium falciparum malaria, 258, 259
geographical spread, 258-259
healers/herbalists (African)
training regimes, 109
modes of entry into herbalist profession, 111-112
African pharmacopoeia of plant remedies excluded poisonous plants, 160-161, 163
how beneficial plants were identified, 195-207
trial and error, 196-202
observation of animals, 202-205
signature plants, 205
and malaria treatment strategy, 281, 304-305
knowledge of anti-inflammatory drugs, 305
herbal medicine
most widely used form of treatment in Africa, 8, 16, 19
in Scotland and England, 34

and modern pharmacology,
155-159
homeopathy
theory of, 232
controversy with medical
scientists, 232
as unethical intervention, 233
Horton, Robin
and traditional African belief
systems, 17, 18
African belief systems as
scientific theory, 49, 50
as a closed predicament,
60-61, 62, 63, 65
immune system
and predisposition to disease,
2-3
and traditional healers, 3
and partial immunity to
malaria, 275, 299-300
incantations
an esoteric practice in traditional African medicine, 4,
7, 12, 192, 220, 228, 229,
230, 269
role of in TAM, 135-137
and placebo effect of, 220, 229-
231
Indian traditional medicine, [see
Ayurveda]
infant mortality (Africa)
and substandard basic
infrastructures, 262-263
inflammation pathology
common factor in many
diseases, 283-284
in asthma, 286-287
in cancer, 287
in sickle cell disease, 257, 288-
289
malaria, 284, 289

and the use of herbal drugs,
285, 304-305
Iroko trees
sacred among many Nigerian
communities, 200
Lambo, Chief J.O.
a traditional healer, 119
and traditional diagnostic
procedures, 119, 125
treating a serious illness, 123
Lambo, T.A.
on the African world view, 45
Last, Murray
on medical culture in Africa,
29, 236
Levy-Bruhl
on mystical orientation of non
literate peoples, 48-49
Luzzatto, Lucio
and G6PD deficiency, 256-258,
302
Makinde, Moses,
on effectiveness of magun, 142-
144
malaria
traditional African approach to
its treatment, 8-9, 274-275,
281, 283, 298, 304
and bacteriostatic agents,
283
and modern medicine, 10, 281,
293
P. falciparum resistance to
modern drugs, 275,
285-282, 291-295
driven by the misuse of
drugs, 303
Ibadan group's formula to
fight resistance, 294-
295
ecologically driven, 14

development of mefloquine, 197, 294
treatment before the colonial period, 246-247, 299-300
and partial immunity in Africans, 248, 251, 252, 254, 257, 261, 274-275, 281, 300
and hypergammaglobin-anaemia, 253
and glucose-6-phosphate dehydrogenase (G6PD) 254-256, 301-302
and sickle cell gene, 253
and P. falciparum malaria, 252-253, 256, 259
and Hb-AS children, 258, 259
WHO control strategies, 249, 250, 298-299
and sickle cell trait, 257-259
and breast-fed infants, 259-261
and PABA deficiency, 262, 263
eradication of, 262
and inflammation, 277-278, 283-284, 305
Maegraith and the pathology of malaria, 277, 278
and cytokine factor, 278
Mbiti, John, 59
modern medicine
and rejection of African traditional medical processes, 34
diagnostic procedures compared to TAM, 119, 183, 209
targets the specific disease, 220, 281, 293
Morris, B.
religion and scientific theories, 68

Nabofa, Michael, 59
and Urhobo divination, 131-133
obo epha
traditional Urhobo diviner, 30, 87
oral tradition
and traditional African medicine, 12, 36-37
Organization of African Unity
adopts WHO definition of traditional healing practices, 16-17
Osuntokun, Professor Benjamin
on household cures for common ailments, 121
pharmacology, modern [also see medicine, modern]
use of drugs to target specific diseases, 155-156, 159, 209, 293
and germ theory of disease, 166
and dosage, 129, 166, 183, 246
digitalis treatment of cardiac disease, 184-185
and bioassay, 185-186
dicourmarol, an anticoagulant, 186
ergot (fungus)medical uses, 187
development of modern drugs from African plants, 188
Calabar bean, 167-181, 183
the therapeutic index, 210, 214
dosage in traditional African medicine, 129, 166, 211, 213-214, 246
and parasite resistance to disease, 69, 302-303
Phyllantus amarus
common anti-inflammatory plant, 121-122

physostigmine, 183
placebo
    defined, 219, 226-227
    as used in modern medicine,
        221, 226
    considered worthless, 227
    and psychoneuroimmuno-logy,
        221
    in clinical trials, 221-226
    effect in TAM, 226
        important element in, 227-
        228
Plasmodium falciparum, 9, 252
    and resistance to anti-malari-als,
        69, 253
    and the cytokine inflammatory
        TNF factor, 261, 278
    malaria parasite, 254-255, 258,
        259
    characteristics of, 297
    and Hb-AS children, 258, 260
    a malaria parasite, 254-255,
        258, 259
Popper, Karl, 61
    on proving scientific theories,
        66-67
    on the verification of metaphy-
        sical theories, 68-69
    and African traditional beliefs,
        66-67
psychoneuroimmunology
    its use in traditional African
        medicine, 3, 94, 242
    and ancestor spirit anger belief,
        34
    brain control and immune
        activity, 49
    stress and illness, 95-96, 100-
        102
sacred trees, 200-201
Salako, L.A, xii

Sapara, Dr. Oguntola
    use of herbs to treat convul-
        sions, 33
Salix alba
    source of aspirin, 267-268
Seyle, Hans
    stress as a factor in disease, 95-
        96, 112
sickle cell disease, 256,
    first reported by Herrick,
        (1910), 256
    (SS) anaemia, 257, 258
    (SC) haemoglobin C, 257
    (SB   +Thal)   sickle   beta
        thalassemia, 257
    crisis, 258
    and Hb-AS sickle cell trait, 258
        and malaria, 258, 289
        and inflammation, 288-289
Sofowora, Professor Abayomi, 118
taboo beliefs and punishment, 137,
        138-141
    many based on hygiene, 140-
        141
    and adultery by women, 141
    magun, adultery by men, 141-
        142
Tavener, John
    and religious revelation, 70
traditional healing systems (Africa)
    two basic types of illness, 7
    response to by Western medi-
        cine, 7-8
    and herbal remedies, 8
    and the African elite, 10
    and Western-trained African
        doctors, 33-34
    and the children of freed
        African slaves, 36
    and treatment of inflamma-tion,
        8, 190-191

herbal treatment of malaria, 247

and serious life threatening illnesses, 52, 123, 125, 126, 164, 229

use of divination as a diagnostic tool, 124, 125, 129-130

Ifa divination, 127-129, 134

Urhobo divination, 130-132

and stress, 126

diagnostic procedures, 120-122

and minor illnesses, 120

fever, headache, 120-121

treated with non poison-ous plants, 165, 166, 190, 192

post-mortem procedures, 124

and oral tradition, 13, 36

advantages of, 37

disease specialists, 126-127

herbalists, 127-129

plants believed to power-ful 135-136

and treatment of fertility and virility, 135-136

uses of poisonous plants, 188-189

Anamirta cocculus (fish poison), 189

Datura strammonium, 189

Gratus strophanthus, 189

and plant nomenclature, 199-200

use of placebo effect in TAM, 226-230, 233

and the use of incantations, 134-135, 136, 229-230

synergistic effects, 231

and the clinical attributes of plants, 232

a constant component in, 235

role in modern medicine in Africa, 237

need to include TAM principles in curricula of medi-cal schools, 240

treatment of malaria

traditional African approach, 8-9, 274-275, 281, 283, 298, 304

and modern medicine, 10, 293

ecologically driven, 14

treatment before the colonial period, 246-247

and partial immunity in Africans, 250, 252, 253, 255, 263, 275, 283, 301-302

and hypergammaglobin-aemia, 253

and WHO Roll Back Malaria, 253, 300

and glucose-6-phosphate dehydrogenase (G6PD), 254-256

and sickle cell gene, 255

and P. falciparum malaria, 254-255

in the partially immune person, 248-249

in the non-immune person, 248

Urhobo divination, 130-132

agbragha apparatus, 132

Urhobo Ughievwen kingdom

Ore, festival of the ancestors, 54

Vane, John

and uses of aspirin, 267

Verger, Pierre Fatumbi

and herbal remedies and incantations, 135

Wiredu, K.
preliterate ways of thought, fn49, 50

witchcraft, 137
defined, 145-146
as social/moral control function, 146, 147
use of esere bean to identify, 167, 168-170172
not studied scientifically, 181

World Health Organization
and treatment of malaria, 10, 251
and definition of traditional healing practices, 15-16, 28
adopted by OAU, 16
its approach to eradicating malaria, 262
Roll Back Malaria, 253, 300
malaria control strategies, 249-251

Yoruba traditional African medicine
magun, 65, 141-144
herbalist, onisegun, 128
and Ifa divination, 128
and herbal plant nomen-clature, 199-20
and signature plants, 205
agbo, 272, 305

Printed in the United States
By Bookmasters